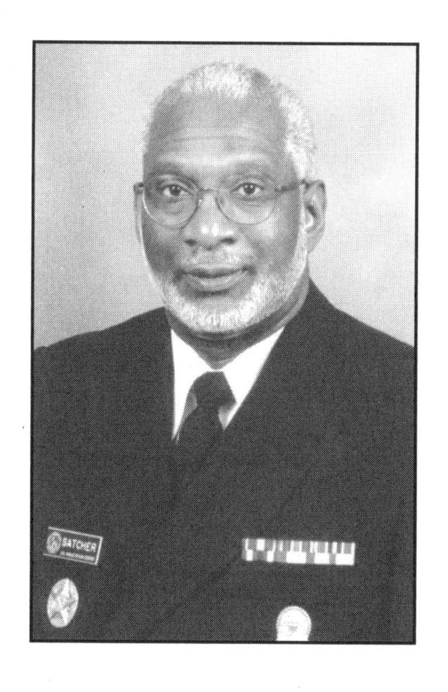

Each year, we learn more about the tremendous health benefits of staying physically active and being properly nourished throughout our lives. The work of scientists, health professionals, and older adult volunteers has greatly increased our knowledge about the aging process and how we can maintain strength, dignity, and independence as we age.

Essential to staying strong and vital during older adulthood is participation in regular strengthening exercises, which help to prevent osteoporosis and frailty by stimulating the growth of muscle and bone. Feeling physically strong also promotes mental and emotional health. Strength training exercises are easy to learn, and have been proven safe and effective through years of thorough research.

Experts at the Centers for Disease Control and Prevention and Tufts University, with the help of older adults, have created this book, ***Growing Stronger: Strength Training for Older Adults*** to help you become stronger and maintain your health and independence. I encourage you to read it carefully and begin using this strength training program as soon as possible. It can make a profound difference in your physical, mental, and emotional health.

Let us aim, as a nation, to Grow Stronger together. To your health—

David Satcher, M.D., Ph.D.
Director, National Center for Primary Care
Morehouse School of Medicine
United States Surgeon General, 1998-2002

STRENGTH TRAINING FOR OLDER ADULTS

growing Stronger

Rebecca A. Seguin, M.S., CSCS[1]
Jacqueline N. Epping, M.Ed.[2]
David Buchner, M.D., M.P.H.[2]
Rina Bloch, M.D.[1]
Miriam E. Nelson, Ph.D.[1]

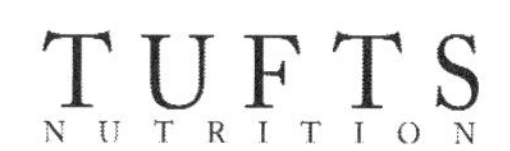

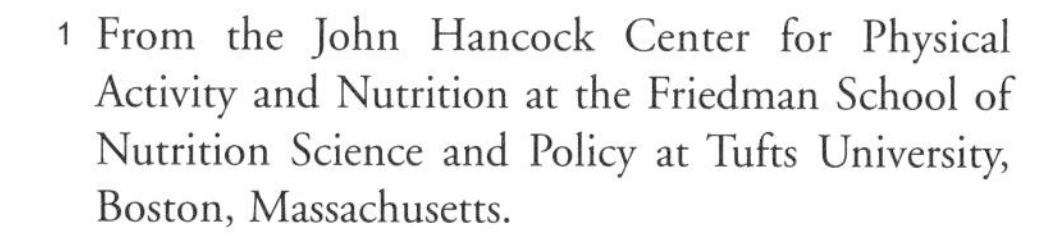
1 From the John Hancock Center for Physical Activity and Nutrition at the Friedman School of Nutrition Science and Policy at Tufts University, Boston, Massachusetts.

2 From the Division of Nutrition and Physical Activity at the Centers for Disease Control and Prevention, Atlanta, Georgia.

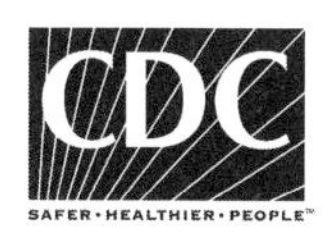

U.S. DEPARTMENT OF HEALTH AND HUMAN SERVICES
Centers for Disease Control and Prevention

Illustrations by Wendy Wray/Morgan Gaynin Inc., NYC.

The PAR-Q test on pages 14 and 15 reprinted from the 1994 revised version of the Physical Activity Readiness Questionnaire (PAR-Q and YOU). The PAR-Q and YOU is a copyrighted, pre-exercise screen owned by the Canadian Society for Exercise Physiology.

This material is based upon work supported by the U.S. Department of Agriculture under agreement number 58-1950-9-001 and the Association of Teachers of Preventive Medicine/Centers for Disease Control and Prevention/Agency for Toxic Substances and Disease Registry cooperative agreement number TS 359-15/16. Any opinions, findings, conclusion, or recommendations expressed in this publication are those of the author(s) and do not necessarily reflect the views of these organizations.

Printed in the United States of America.

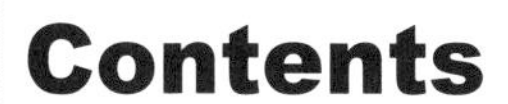

Contents

An Important Caution

The **Growing Stronger** exercise program is based on extensive scientific research. The book contains detailed instructions and safety cautions, and you are urged to read them carefully. If you are under a physician's care for a medical condition, discuss this program with him or her before you start. Remember that regular medical checkups are essential for your health and well-being. While this book can serve as your guide to growing stronger and becoming more physically active, it cannot replace the advice of a health care professional who knows you personally.

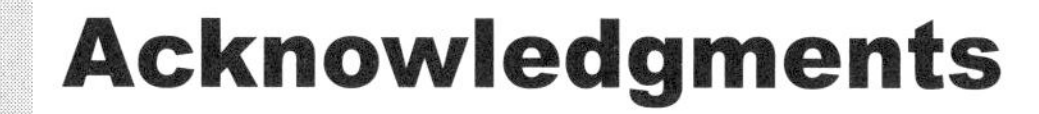

Acknowledgments

This book would not have been possible without the time and assistance of our Peer Advisory Board members, Sister Mary Patrice, Al, Dorothy, and Helen. These individuals unselfishly donated their time; some provided their expertise and others shared their experiences of living with arthritis as well as starting—and continuing—a strength training program. Several of the Peer Advisory Board members were volunteers in our research center for arthritis studies, which are the foundation for the **Growing Stronger** program. We are so grateful for their help with this project.

Before completing this book, we worked with another set of volunteers whose insight was invaluable to the success of this book. These individuals had no previous experience with strength training, and they volunteered to try the **Growing Stronger** program on their own and provide feed-back on numerous aspects of the book and exercises. We wish to extend our sincere gratitude to these volunteers and to the countless others like them who have made enormous contributions to keep scientific research moving forward and without whom our work would not be possible.

Several of our colleagues at Tufts and elsewhere contributed to the success of this project. Many thanks to Drs. Irwin Rosenberg, Ronenn Roubenoff, Kristin Baker, and Bess Marcus for their encouragement as well as their personal contribution to the body of research that helped form the basis for the **Growing Stronger** program. Jennifer Layne, M.S., CSCS, donated her time to review the exercise program. Her expertise and experience was invaluable. Finally, to all of the members of the Nutrition, Exercise Physiology and Sarcopenia Laboratory as well as our other colleagues at Tufts University and the Centers for Disease Control and Prevention, we are grateful for your feedback about this book and for your continued support.

We had the benefit of collaborating with several talented individuals for different aspects of this book. We wish to acknowledge Jennifer Ackerman for her editorial genius and thoughtful contribution to reshaping certain sections of the book. Thank you to Wendy Wray for the wonderful illustrations and to Ilana Rosenberg for her creative energy and diligent work on the design of this book.

preface

An Exercise Program for You

In choosing to read this book, you have taken the first step on a journey toward greater strength and vitality. **Growing Stronger** was written for you—the older adult who wants to grow stronger, healthier, more active, and more independent. You may be inactive or only mildly active at the moment. You may know that regular exercise is important for your health and well-being and want to get started on a program of physical activity. But you may feel that you don't have the necessary information. Perhaps you are concerned that because of your age or health problems physical activity may not be safe for you. Or perhaps you have had trouble finding or staying with a suitable program.

This book gives you a safe, simple, and highly effective exercise program based on the principles of strength training. Studies at laboratories around the world have shown that strength training benefits women and men of all ages and all levels of fitness. According to *Physical Activity and Health: A Report of the Surgeon General* (1996), experts agree that aerobic activities should be supplemented with strength-developing exercises at least twice per week.

These activities will help you:

- build strength
- maintain bone density
- improve balance, coordination, and mobility
- reduce your risk of falling
- maintain independence in performing activities of daily life.

Strength training requires little time and minimal equipment. And it's safe, even for people with health problems. The strength training "prescription" featured here—the motivational tips, safety precautions, and specific exercises—was developed at the Nutrition, Exercise Physiology and Sarcopenia Laboratory at Tufts University. Whatever your age, medical condition, or current level of activity, you are likely a perfect candidate for this gentle but powerful program.

This book gives you all the tools you need to succeed in this exciting program. It introduces you to the many advantages of strength training—boosts in strength, energy, and vitality and the role it plays in helping to prevent and treat such chronic diseases as arthritis and osteoporosis. It helps you decide whether these exercises are safe for you or whether you need to consult with your doctor first. It offers a program tailored to your needs, with step-by-step instructions on getting started, staying on track, and growing stronger and healthier as you age. At the end of the book is a 12-week workbook in which you can record and gauge your progress and celebrate your success.

The goal of this program is to help you make strength training a lifelong habit. By doing so, you will be on your way to a strong, independent, and vibrant life!

chapter 1 The Power of Strength Training

For many older adults, growing older seems to involve an inevitable loss of strength, energy, and vigor. But it need not be so. The frailty and decreased energy we associate with aging, such as difficulty walking for distances, climbing stairs, or carrying groceries, are largely due to muscle loss. This muscle loss results mainly from inactivity. The old saying is true when it comes to muscle: "Use it or lose it."

One of the best ways to keep muscles healthy and strong is through exercises called strength training—sometimes known as weight lifting or resistance training. Studies at Tufts University have shown that strength training is one of the best ways to fight the weakness and frailty that can come with age. Done regularly, strength training builds bone and muscle and helps to preserve strength, independence, and energy. These exercises are safe and effective for women and men of all ages, including those who are not in perfect health. In fact, people with health concerns—such as arthritis or heart disease—often benefit the most from an exercise program that includes lifting weights a few times each week.

Strength training can also reduce the signs and symptoms of many diseases and chronic conditions in the following ways:

- *Arthritis*—Reduces pain and stiffness, and increases strength and flexibility.
- *Diabetes*—Improves glycemic control.
- *Osteoporosis*—Builds bone density and reduces risk for falls.
- *Heart disease*—Reduces cardiovascular risk by improving lipid profile and overall fitness.
- *Obesity*—Increases metabolism, which helps burn more calories and helps with long-term weight control.
- *Back pain*—Strengthens back and abdominal muscles to reduce stress on the spine.

Strength training, when done with regular aerobic exercise, can also have a major effect on a person's mental and emotional health. Studies have shown that people who exercise regularly sleep better; they sleep more deeply and longer and awaken less often. Strength training exercises can also reduce depression and boost self-confidence and self-esteem, and improve your sense of well-being.

The exercises that make up the **Growing Stronger** strength training program have been widely tested on healthy individuals and people with chronic but stable medical concerns. No matter how old you are, you do not have to get weaker with age. Strength training can help you stay vital, strong, and independent throughout your life. Start the **Growing Stronger** program and make it a regular part of your life so you can begin enjoying the many physical and emotional benefits of strength training today.

chapter 2

Making Change

Introducing any major change into our daily lives can be very challenging. Starting an exercise program is like setting off on a journey; it requires a step-by-step approach. When making any major lifestyle changes, most people go through 5 stages, as defined by the transtheoretical model: pre-contemplation, contemplation, preparation, action, and maintenance.

CONTEMPLATION—GETTING MOTIVATED

By reading this book, you have already moved beyond pre-contemplation, which is the stage in which you're not yet thinking about strength training. In contemplation, you are intrigued by what you have heard about strength training. Reading about the health benefits of these exercises or hearing about them from a friend or doctor has stimulated your interest in starting the program yourself. At this stage, you work on getting motivated, thinking about your goals, and asking yourself what you want to get out of the program. This is also the time to address possible obstacles and find ways to overcome them.

PREPARATION—STARTING YOUR JOURNEY

You are ready to take action once you have thought about your motivations and goals for strength training. At this stage, you take steps to prepare for a new exercise program. You set aside the physical space needed to do the exercises and buy any equipment you may need. You look at your schedule to see where strength training might fit in and set specific exercise days and times.

ACTION—ADOPTING THE PROGRAM

At this exciting stage, you are learning the exercises and doing them 2 or 3 times per week. You are beginning to see the results of your work. You notice physical changes and find that your clothes fit a little better and that you feel stronger, more energetic, and happier. Technically, the action stage continues as long as you are engaged in the program. But after about 6 months of doing the exercises, you will have moved to the maintenance stage.

MAINTENANCE—STAYING ON TRACK

This is the stage when strength training becomes a way of life. When you reach this point, there's a good chance that you find it hard to imagine *not* doing your exercises. You find them empowering and enjoyable and want to continue them because they make you feel stronger and more upbeat, independent, and vital. You may find that you're taking up activities you had stopped doing years ago—gardening, golfing, dancing, or canoeing. As you progress, you may also add new strengthening exercises to your routine and new activities to your life.

Here's a timetable for moving through the first three stages of change:

Days 1–5: Read this book and set goals (contemplation)

Days 6–10: Buy equipment and set an exercise schedule (preparation)

Days 11–12: Start the program (action)

For some people, one stage flows easily and naturally into the next in a short period of time with few major problems. But many of us get hung up at one stage or another. Keep in mind that it often takes several tries to change one's daily routine. Stay with it—you'll find that the effort pays off in ways you never imagined!

chapter 3

Getting Motivated

If you want to make a positive, lasting change in your life, it helps to spend some time thinking about what motivates you. What are your reasons for wanting to strength train? What are your personal goals? What obstacles might stop you and how might you overcome them? It's also a good idea to visualize your success and consider how you might celebrate your achievements.

SETTING GOALS

Thirty years ago, a British doctor put together a list of the reasons why people choose to exercise. Look at the reasons listed below and see which of them match your motivations:

Pleasure. People often enjoy strength-training exercises; they find them easier than aerobic workouts and love the results.

Health and fitness benefits. Strength training can increase muscle mass and bone density. It makes you feel strong and energized, relieves stress and depression, and gives you a better night's sleep. It can also help prevent the onset of certain chronic diseases or ease their symptoms.

Improvements in appearance. Lifting weights firms the body, trims fat, and can boost metabolism by as much as 15 percent, which helps control your weight.

Social opportunities. Exercising with friends or family gives you a chance to visit and chat while you work out.

Thrills. People who start strength training later in life often find that they are willing and able to try new, exciting activities, such as parasailing, windsurfing, or kayaking.

Chapter 4, "Starting Your Journey," includes worksheets on setting your own short-term and long-term goals. These worksheets will help you personalize the benefits of the program.

ELIMINATING OBSTACLES

While thinking about your motivations, you will want to consider possible obstacles and plan ways to overcome them. The most common barriers seem to be:

Time. For many of us, being too busy is the big obstacle. How can we find a few times each week to exercise? You might consider combining strength training with another activity or with a social visit. Try scheduling your sessions during a lunch-hour break or during a favorite television program.

Instead of going out to lunch, lift weights with a good friend or family member. The half hour or so that you spend watching the evening news is a perfect time to sneak in a whole workout.

Fatigue. It's a proven fact that strength training gives you more energy; it also makes other daily activities easier.

Age or fitness. If you think you're too old or out of shape to lift weights, rest assured. People have successfully started strength training in their 70s, 80s, and even 90s, and you can too! The same goes for people who are not active. You will need to start slowly and follow basic safety rules. But there is no such thing as being too old or out of shape to benefit from this program.

Health concerns. If you have a health problem, you should talk to your doctor before you start any exercise program. But chances are that your condition will not stop you from strength training. In fact, you may be among those who gain the most from this form of exercise.

VISUALIZING SUCCESS

The ticket to success is believing in yourself and your ability to overcome barriers and reach your goals. Visualization, a process of "training" the mind, is one of the best ways to build self-confidence. It involves imagining that you are accomplishing desired changes or goals and successfully completing each step in a given activity. As a result, you can create, modify, or strengthen brain pathways that prepare your muscles for the activity. Visualization is useful in many areas of life, from avoiding stress to performing well during competition. You may find it a powerful tool as you begin this program.

First, it's a good idea to define your personal goals so you can apply them during the visualization process. For instance, if you hope to start walking the golf course again or spend longer hours gardening, you might establish these as your specific goals. The technique is simple, but you will need to practice to make it work well for you. It does not require equipment and does not cost money, but it does take time and focus.

CELEBRATE YOUR ACHIEVEMENTS

Making any major lifestyle change can be challenging. Celebrating your success is a great way to motivate yourself

USING VISUALIZATION

1. Identify the goal you want to visualize—for example, taking a sunrise foliage hike in the woods with your spouse, best friend, or grandchildren.
2. Find a comfortable place to sit and relax.
3. Eliminate all distractions—turn off the phone and television. Close your eyes and focus on feeling relaxed. Free your mind of intruding thoughts.
4. Now, imagine yourself waking up a little before sunrise on a Sunday morning. Picture the place in your mind—the sites, sounds, and smells such as the warm aroma of coffee percolating. Picture yourself eating a healthy breakfast and getting dressed for your hike. You step outdoors and feel the cool, crisp air and smell the familiar scent of fallen leaves. Imagine yourself chatting with close family or friends as you start the hike. Listen to the crackling of leaves and twigs under your feet as the sun begins to rise.
5. Take a moment to feel the pleasure and serenity of this hike with loved ones. Imagine the sunlight is trickling through the trees as you're walking. The temperature is rising, and the sun and exercise are warming your body.
6. Finally, visualize yourself reaching the destination of your hike, feeling exhilarated and energized. You're high enough so that you can see above the trees to the valley below. Everyone gasps at the breathtaking views of the leaves' changing beauty.

to keep with the program. This may be as important as setting goals and visualizing success. Make sure that you reward yourself well when you accomplish one of your short-term or long-term goals!

Cause for Celebration

Here are some ideas for celebrating your success:

- Make plans with friends to see a movie or go hiking.
- Buy yourself new workout clothes or shoes.
- Go on a weekend getaway.
- Treat yourself to a new piece of exercise equipment.
- Plan a dinner at your favorite restaurant.
- Get tickets to your favorite theater production or athletic event.
- Pamper yourself with a massage, manicure, or pedicure.
- Enroll in a class, such as ballroom dancing, yoga, or pottery making.

chapter 4 Starting Your Journey: 6 Simple Steps

Now that you have thought about your own motivations for strength training, you are ready to prepare for the program. Follow these simple steps:

STEP 1: DETERMINE IF STRENGTH TRAINING IS SAFE FOR YOU

It's important to talk to your doctor before beginning any exercise program if you have health concerns. Chronic health conditions should not stop you from strength training. It's likely that you will still be able to take part in this program if you have arthritis, osteoporosis, diabetes, congestive heart failure, or have recently suffered a heart attack.

First it's important to find out whether or not you need to speak with your doctor before you can safely start the program. The Physical Activity Readiness Questionnaire —known as the PAR-Q—is on the next two pages. These questions will help you get started.

Physical Activity Readiness
Questionnaire—PAR-Q
(revised 2002)

PAR-Q & YOU

(A Questionnaire for People Aged 15-69)

Regular physical activity is fun and healthy, and increasingly more people are starting to become more active every day. Being more active is very safe for most people. However, some people should check with their doctor before they start becoming much more physically active.

If you are planning to become much more physically active than you are now, start by answering the seven questions in the box below. If you are between the ages of 15 and 69, the PAR-Q will tell you if you should check with your doctor before you start. If you are over 69 years of age, and you are not used to being very active, check with your doctor.

Common sense is your best guide when you answer these questions. Please read the questions carefully and answer each one honestly: check YES or NO.

YES	NO	
☐	☐	1. Has your doctor ever said that you have a heart condition and that you should only do physical activity recommended by a doctor?
☐	☐	2. Do you feel pain in your chest when you do physical activity?
☐	☐	3. In the past month, have you had chest pain when you were not doing physical activity?
☐	☐	4. Do you lose your balance because of dizziness or do you ever lose consciousness?
☐	☐	5. Do you have a bone or joint problem (for example, back, knee, or hip) that could be made worse by a change in your physical activity?
☐	☐	6 . Is your doctor currently prescribing drugs (for example water pills) for your blood pressure or heart condition?
☐	☐	7. Do you know of any other reason why you should not do physical activity?

IF YOU ANSWERED

YES to one or more questions

Talk with your doctor by phone or in person BEFORE you start becoming much more physically active or BEFORE you have a fitness appraisal. Tell your doctor about the PAR-Q and which questions you answered YES.

- You may be able to do any activity you want—as long as you start slowly and build up gradually. Or, you may need to restrict your activities to those which are safe for you. Talk with your doctor about the kinds of physical activities you wish to participate in and follow his/her advice.
- Find out which community programs are safe and helpful for you.

No to all questions

If you answered NO honestly to *all* PAR-Q questions, you can be reasonably sure that you can:

- start becoming much more physically active—begin slowly and build up gradually. This is the safest and easiest way to go.
- take part in a fitness appraisal—this is an excellent way to determine your basic fitness so that you can plan the best way for you to live actively.

DELAY BECOMING MUCH MORE ACTIVE:

- if you are not feeling well because of a temporary illness such as a cold or fever—wait until you feel better;

  or
- if you are or may be pregnant—talk to your doctor before you start becoming more active.

Please Note: If your health changes so that you then answer YES to any of the above questions, tell your fitness or health care professional. Ask whether you should change your physical activity plan.

Informed Use of the PAR-Q: The Canadian Society for Exercise Physiology, Health Canada, and their agents assume no liability for persons who undertake physical activity, and if in doubt after completing this questionnaire, consult your doctor prior to activity.

You should get approval from your doctor if you answered “yes” to one or more questions on the PAR-Q or if you are over the age of 69. Answering “yes” or being older than 69 simply means that you should discuss the program with your doctor before getting started. You can get started right away if you honestly answered “no” to all of the questions and are between the ages of 15–69.

IF YOU HAVE ONE OR MORE CHRONIC DISEASES, KEEP THESE THINGS IN MIND

- Speak with your doctor before starting any new exercise program–you may need a physical examination.
- Stay in touch with your doctor about your exercise program and your health.
- Never exercise if you have a health condition that is unstable or serious, you have new symptoms, or your doctor recommends against it.

STEP 2: FIND OUT HOW FIT AND STRONG YOU ARE NOW?

Before you start this program, answer the questions on the next two pages in the worksheet **How Fit and Strong Are You Now?** Try returning to them again after you have been strength training for 3, 6, and 12 months. This will help you see how useful the program has been to you.

Record your score for each question in the "start" column and then add all of the scores together. Answer the questions again at the 3-, 6-, and 12-month marks. Add up each score and compare it with previous scores. An increase of even a point or two from the last test is a great improvement. Remember, your score may stay the same or even decrease if you have not stayed on the program for any reason—say, illness or injury. Don't be discouraged—just try to get back on track.

How Fit and Strong Are You Now?

RARELY (1 POINT) SOMETIMES (2 POINTS) USUALLY (3 POINTS) ALWAYS (4 POINTS)

MOBILITY AND DAILY ACTIVITIES:	START	3 MONTHS	6 MONTHS	9 MONTHS	12 MONTHS
1. I find it easy to walk up or down two or more flights of stairs.					
2. I have no trouble taking out the trash.					
3. I do housework such as vacuuming and dusting on my own without difficulty.					
4. I can easily lift a gallon of milk (8 lbs).					
5. I can easily walk a mile.					
6. I have no trouble reaching into high cupboards or reaching down to pick up something from the floor.					
7. I do not have trouble doing outdoor work such as mowing the lawn, raking leaves, or gardening.					
TOTAL					

How Fit and Strong Are You Now?

RARELY (1 POINT) SOMETIMES (2 POINTS) USUALLY (3 POINTS) ALWAYS (4 POINTS)

MOOD, ENERGY LEVEL AND MENTAL HEALTH	START	3 MONTHS	6 MONTHS	9 MONTHS	12 MONTHS
1. I feel younger than my age.					
2. I feel independent.					
3. I feel energetic.					
4. I live an active life.					
5. I feel strong.					
6. I feel healthy.					
7. I am as active as other people my age.					
TOTAL FROM THIS PAGE					
TOTAL PREVIOUS PAGE					
GRAND TOTAL					

Evaluating your score

15–29 POINTS: Low fitness level, with a lot of room for improvement in mobility, ability to complete daily tasks, and mood and mental health.

30–39 POINTS: Low-to-moderate fitness level, with room for improvement in most of the above areas.

40–49 POINTS: Moderate fitness level, with room for improvement in some of the above areas.

50+ POINTS: Advanced fitness level; strength training will improve and maintain fitness.

STEP 3: DEFINE YOUR GOALS

When taking on any challenge, it's a good idea to define your goals. You should identify what you want to accomplish and how you will carry out your plan. This is important when making positive change and will help you succeed.

Before starting this program, set short-term and long-term goals. These goals should be **S-M-A-R-T**:

S — **SPECIFIC**
M — **MEASURABLE**
A — **ATTAINABLE**
R — **RELEVANT**
T — **TIME-BASED**

For instance:

- A **SPECIFIC** short-term goal may be to start strength training; the long-term goal may be easing the symptoms of arthritis, improving balance, or controlling your weight.
- This goal is easily **MEASURABLE:** Have you or have you not begun the program?
- Indeed, this is an **ATTAINABLE** goal, as long as your doctor approves.
- And this goal is certainly **RELEVANT** to living a long, healthy life.
- Your goal should be **TIME-BASED:** you should read this

book within 5 days; buy the equipment you need and set your exercise schedule within the next 5 days. Start the program within the next 2 to 3 days.

The goals and timeframe are entirely up to you. You may want to focus your long-term goals on improving a specific health condition, such as reducing pain from arthritis, controlling diabetes, increasing bone density to help combat osteoporosis, or increasing muscle mass to help with balance or weight control. Or your goal may be to bowl or play tennis, or perhaps, to do all of your own chores, such as cleaning windows or vacuuming. Your success depends on setting goals that are truly important to you—and possessing a strong desire to achieve them.

GOAL-SETTING WORKSHEET #1:
IDENTIFYING YOUR SHORT-TERM GOALS

Identify at least two or three of your own short-term goals. If you have more goals, write them down now. Remember that each goal should be **S-M-A-R-T**—**S**pecific, **M**easurable, **A**ttainable, **R**elevant, and **T**ime-based. Setting these short-term goals will help motivate you to make the program a regular part of your life.

MY SHORT-TERM GOALS

Examples:

- I will talk to my doctor about starting this program.
- I will buy the equipment I need and get ready to exercise within 2 weeks.
- I will look at my calendar and schedule 2 or 3 45-minute blocks of time for exercise each week.
- I will invite my spouse/friend/family member to join me in these exercises.

SMART

MY PERSONAL SHORT-TERM GOALS:

1.

2.

3.

4.

5.

GOAL-SETTING WORKSHEET #2:
IDENTIFYING YOUR LONG-TERM GOALS

Identify at least two or three long-term goals. If you have more goals, write them down now. Are there activities that you want to do more easily over the long term? Are there things that you haven't done in some time that you want to try again? Listing these goals will help you stay with the program, see your progress, and enjoy your success. (Don't forget to use the **S-M-A-R-T** technique.)

MY LONG-TERM GOALS

Examples:

- I will do each exercise 2 or 3 times each week. Within 3 months, I will do each exercise with 5-lb weights.
- After 12 weeks of the program, I will take the stairs instead of the elevator.
- I will be able to walk to the store or office.
- I will do my own vacuuming.
- I will play golf.
- I will reduce some of the pain and stiffness from arthritis.

SMART

MY PERSONAL LONG-TERM GOALS:

1.

2.

3.

4.

5.

STEP 4: GET EQUIPMENT

Strength training requires little special equipment, but there are a few basic necessities:

A sturdy chair and exercise space

Find a strong, stable chair that does not rock or sway when you sit in it or move when you stand up from it. When you sit in the chair, your knees should be at a 90-degree angle and your feet should be flat on the ground. If the chair is too high, find one with shorter legs; if it's too low, try putting a pillow or a folded blanket on the seat to give you a slight boost.

For your exercise space, choose an open area, preferably carpeted, with at least enough space for your chair and ample room to walk around it. Carpeting will stop the chair from sliding. On bare floor, put your chair against the wall. If want to exercise to music or while watching television, plan your space accordingly.

Good shoes

Good shoes are essential for any exercise. For strength training, try athletic shoes with good support, such as walking, running, or cross-training sneakers. The sole should be rubber, but not too thick, because fat soles may cause you to trip. If you don't already have the right shoes, you can find them at sporting goods, discount, and department stores.

Comfortable clothing

Wear loose, cool clothing that breathes well during exercise—for example, a cotton T-shirt and cotton shorts or pants. If you want to buy new workout clothes, look for materials that absorb moisture and that you feel comfortable in.

Dumbbells (hand-held weights) and ankle weights

You can do the first part of the exercise program without weights. You will need dumbbells and ankle weights as you get stronger and add new exercises. It's a good idea to buy these before you begin strength training or soon after you start, so that you'll have them when you're ready. You should buy a set of 2 dumbbells in each of the following weights:

WOMEN	MEN
2 pounds	3 pounds
3 pounds	5 pounds
5 pounds	8 pounds

The best ankle weights for this program are the adjustable type. These let you add weight gradually until you reach as much as 10 or 20 pounds per leg.

You have several options when buying equipment:

Options	Benefits	Drawbacks
Newspaper, want-ads	Inexpensive	Used; can't return
Sporting goods store	Can test product	Slightly more expensive
Mail order	Convenient	Shipping is costly

Some stores and mail-order companies offer specials that include a set of 2-, 3-, and 5-pound weights at discounted prices. This is a good starter kit; later you can buy sets with heavier weights. Discount department stores as well as sporting good stores should have a good selection of dumbbells and adjustable ankle weights.

STORAGE CONTAINER

For safety reasons, consider storing your weights in a floor-level cupboard or in a container such as a wooden box or canvas bag—preferably on a cart with wheels so you can move them easily. You can usually buy storage containers and wheeled carts at local department and discount stores. If you do not use a cart, try to keep your weights in the area where you exercise so you don't have to move them a lot. Also, remember to store weights away from children and in a place where people will not trip over them.

STEP 5: SCHEDULE YOUR EXERCISE

Look at your schedule to see where strength training may best fit in—perhaps on weekday mornings before work or during your favorite evening TV show. There are no rules about the best time to exercise. But keep in mind that you should exercise on three non-consecutive days of the week (say, Monday, Wednesday, and Friday; or Tuesday, Thursday, Saturday). This gives your muscles a proper rest. You can also try doing lower body exercises one day and then upper body exercises the next. This way, you will avoid overworking the same muscle groups.

Put your scheduled strength-training appointments on your calendar and keep them faithfully, just as you would a doctor's appointment. You might also try to find an exercise partner who can join you for your scheduled sessions. Exercising with a friend will help you adhere to your routine and keep you motivated.

Here are some tips on scheduling exercise:

- Consider what days best suit your schedule, given your other commitments.
- Pick a time of day when you most enjoy exercising. Some people like to exercise first thing in the morning; others are more motivated in the evening or afternoon.
- Write your first exercise appointments on your calendar. After your first 2 or 3 sessions, decide whether your selected days and times work well for you. If they don't, look at your schedule again and try to find better times.

STEP 6: EXERCISE SAFE AND SMART

At times, you will not feel like exercising. This is true for everyone. If you're just feeling a little tired or low on energy, go ahead and try to exercise. The workout will likely boost your energy level and your mood. However, if you're not feeling well—if you think you might be getting sick, coming down with a cold or the flu; or if you have any kind of pain or swelling—take a break from exercising and, if necessary, contact your doctor. Your health and safety are the top priorities.

The reasons listed below are good cause to take a day off from strength training. Be cautious—if you're not sure whether you're well enough to exercise, take a break and see how you feel the next day.

REFRAIN FROM EXERCISING OR CHECK WITH YOUR DOCTOR FIRST IF YOU HAVE:

- A cold, flu, or infection accompanied by fever.
- Significantly more fatigue than usual.
- A swollen or painful muscle or joint.
- Any new or undiagnosed symptom.
- Chest pain or irregular, rapid, or fluttery heartbeat.
- Shortness of breath.
- A hernia with symptoms.
- Been advised by your doctor not to exert yourself for a given period of time due to illness, surgery, etc.

Listen to your body. You will know when you're well enough to handle a workout and when you need to take a day off or see your doctor, as you get used to your exercise program.

chapter 5 Getting Stronger: A 3-Part Program

The strength-training program outlined in this book has three phases:

- **Part I** strengthens your body slowly and gently, using only your own body weight
- **Part II** introduces dumbbells and ankle weights to increase strength
- **Part III** adds variety with new ways to boost your strength even more.

The exercises in this program were devised in a research laboratory at Tufts University. The exercises are safe and effective. They are designed to strengthen all of the major muscle groups in the upper body (shoulders, upper arms, back, chest, and abdomen) and in the lower body (hips, thighs, knees, lower legs, and ankles). They also target muscles affected by osteoarthritis, particularly in the shoulders, hands, hips, and knees.

The exercises involve lifting a heavy load—either your own body weight or a dumbbell or ankle weight—by raising the weight (to a count of two to four) and then lowering it (to a count of four) in a smooth, fluid motion. The full motion is then repeated 10 times to make a full "set," or group of repetitions.

Here's a timetable for going through the three parts of the program:

Part I: Weeks 1 – 2

Part II: Weeks 3 – 6

Part III: Weeks 7 +

Once you have done the exercises in Part I two or three times a week for at least two weeks, you can safely move on to Part II. Do the exercises in Part II two or three times a week for four weeks before you move on to the exercises described in Part III.

Chapter 7 includes a 12-week workbook. Start keeping a record in this workbook when you begin strength training. It will help you monitor your progress and stay on track with the program. Research studies show that record-keeping helps people stay with strength training over the long term.

Make sure that you are doing each exercise safely and properly with the full range of motion. Also, make sure that you stretch after each workout and breathe regularly throughout the exercises—don't hold your breath!

WARM-UP

PART I:

4 EXERCISES FOR GETTING STARTED

This first part of your exercise program starts you on your journey to greater strength, balance, and coordination. This part is gentle and requires no special equipment so it can serve as an anchor program. You only need a chair and a wall. It's helpful (but not necessary) to have a mirror so you can check your form during the exercises.

Later, once you have moved to Part II or III, if you're not feeling well or if you're away from home, you can do these exercises to keep up with your program.

Exercise Tip

Remember to breathe regularly throughout each exercise. This will help keep blood and oxygen flowing to your working muscles.

WARM-UP

5-MINUTE WALK

Walk for 5 minutes to get your muscles warm and loose for strength training. You can walk outside if weather permits, inside around the house, or on a treadmill if you have one. Walking will help direct blood flow to your muscles and get your body ready for exercise. Warming up is important for preventing injury. It also helps you get the most benefit from the exercise, because flexible, warm muscles respond better to the challenge of lifting weights.

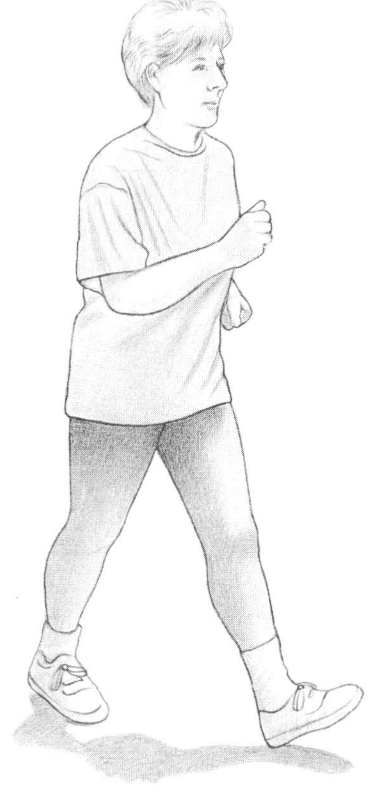

You can also use a bike, rowing machine, stair stepper or other piece of aerobic equipment to warm up.

EXERCISE 1

SQUATS

A great exercise for strengthening hips, thighs, and buttocks. Before long, you'll find that walking, jogging, and climbing stairs are a snap!

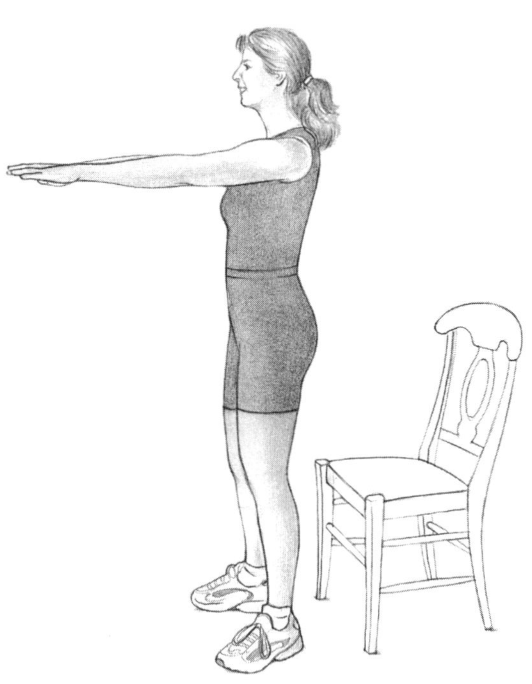

1. Stand directly in front of a sturdy chair. Your feet should be slightly more than shoulder-width apart. Extend your arms so that they are parallel to the ground.
2. Place your weight more on your heels than on the balls of your feet. Bend your knees as you lower your buttocks towards the chair in a slow, controlled motion, while you count to 4.

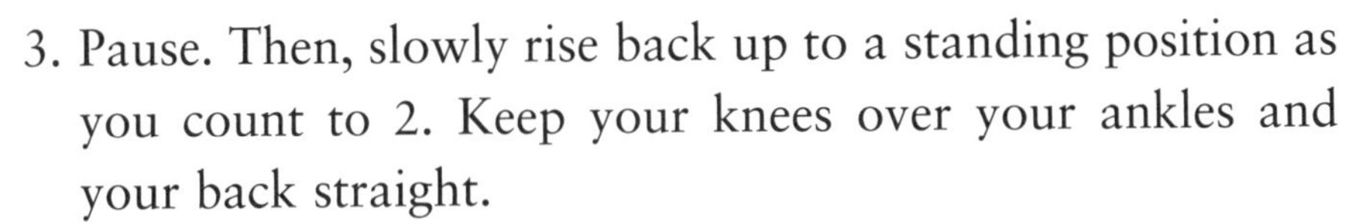

3. Pause. Then, slowly rise back up to a standing position as you count to 2. Keep your knees over your ankles and your back straight.

Repeat the squat ten times. This equals 1 set. Rest for about 1 minute. Then complete a second set of 10 squats.

EXERCISE 1

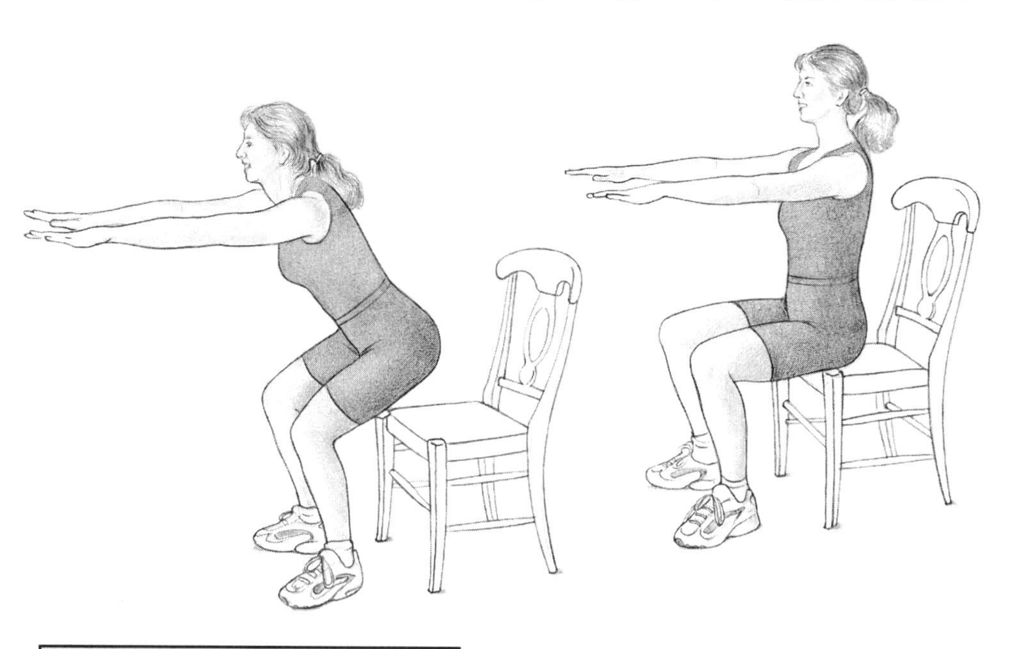

MAKE SURE YOU

Don't sit down too quickly.

Don't lean your weight too far forward or onto your toes when standing up.

Note 1

Start off by using your hands for support if this exercise is too difficult. Also, if you can't sit all the way down or if you feel pain or discomfort, place a couple of pillows on the chair or only squat down 4 to 6 inches.

Note 2

Make sure that your knees NEVER come forward past your toes—this can put stress on the knee joint. This will also help you use your hip muscles more as you rise to a standing position.

EXERCISE 2

WALL PUSH-UPS

This exercise is a modified version of the push-up you may have done years ago in physical education classes. It is easier than a push-up and you don't need to get down on the floor—but it will help to strengthen your arms, shoulders, and chest.

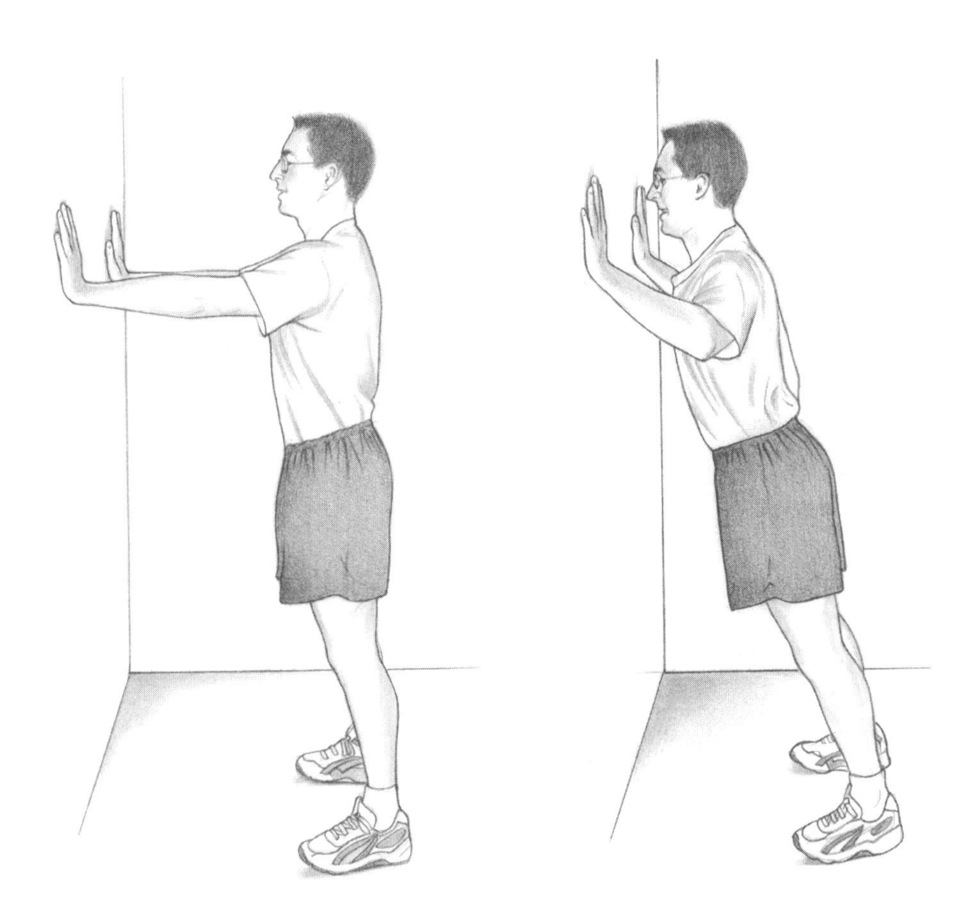

EXERCISE 2

1. Find a wall that is clear of any objects such as wall hangings and windows. Stand a little farther than arm's length from the wall. Face the wall, lean your body forward and place your palms flat against the wall at about shoulder height and shoulder-width apart.
2. Bend your elbows as you lower your upper body toward the wall in a slow, controlled motion as you count to 4. Keep your feet planted.
3. Pause. Then, slowly push yourself back until your arms are straight as you count to 4. Make sure you don't lock your elbows.

Repeat the wall push-up 10 times for 1 set. Rest for about 1 minute. Then do a second set of 10 wall push-ups.

MAKE SURE YOU

Keep your hands planted on the wall for each set.

Don't round or arch your back.

EXERCISE 3

TOE STANDS

If a walk in the park no longer seems easy or enjoyable, the toe stand exercise is for you! It will help make that stroll in the park fun and relaxing by strengthening your calves and ankles and restoring stability and balance.

1. Stand with your feet shoulder-width apart near a counter or sturdy chair. Use the chair or counter for balance.
2. Slowly push up as far as you can onto the balls of your feet as you count to 4. Hold this position for 2 to 4 seconds.
3. Then, slowly lower your heels back to the floor as you count to 4.

Repeat 10 toe stands for 1 set. Rest for about 1 minute. Then complete a second set of 10 toe stands.

MAKE SURE YOU

Don't lean on the counter or chair—use it for balance only.

Breathe regularly throughout the exercise.

EXERCISE 3

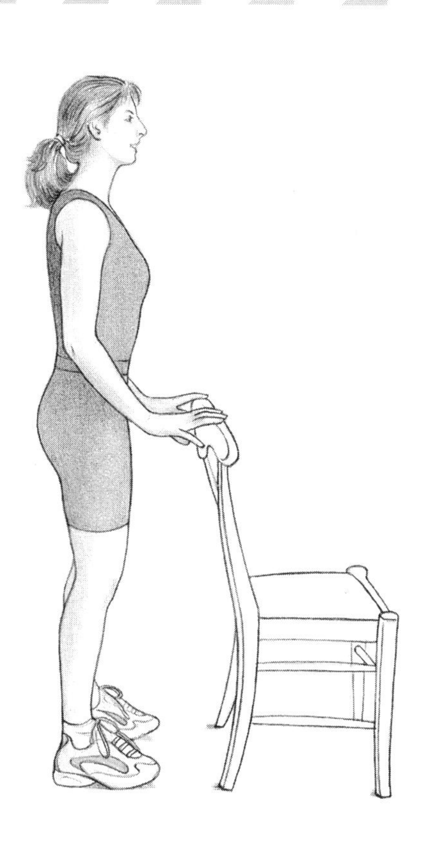

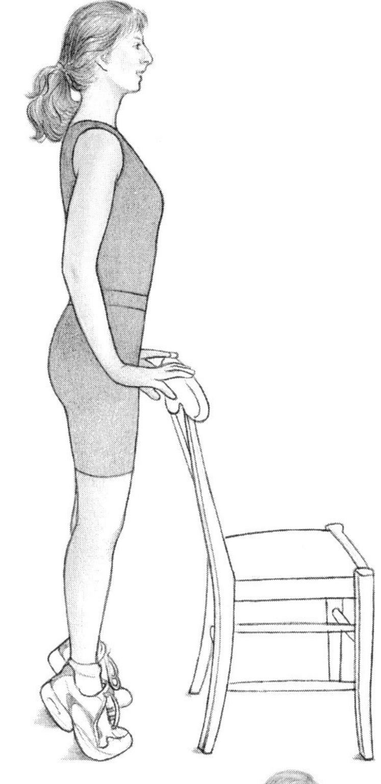

Advanced Move

Doing this toe stand exercise on a staircase will increase its intensity.

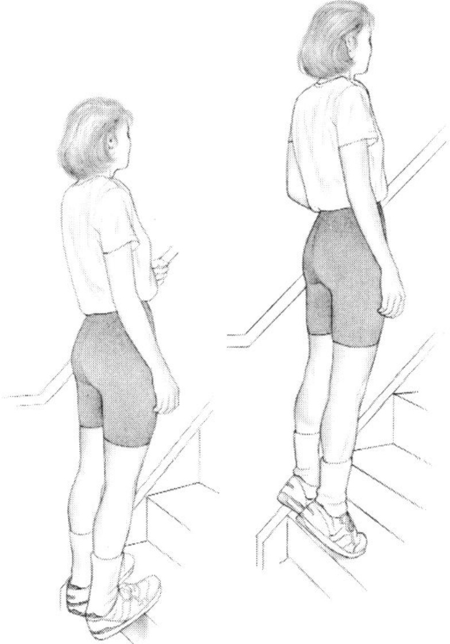

EXERCISE 4

FINGER MARCHING

In this exercise, you'll let your fingers, hands, and arms do the walking. This will help strengthen your upper body and your grip. It will also increase the flexibility of your arms, back, and shoulders.

Stand or sit forward in a chair with your feet on the floor. Your feet should be shoulder-width apart.

Movement 1: Imagine there is a wall directly in front of you. Slowly walk your fingers up the wall until your arms are above your head. Hold your arms overhead while wiggling your fingers for about 10 seconds. Then slowly walk them back down.

Movement 2: Next, try to touch your hands behind your back. If you can, reach for the opposite elbow with each hand—or get as close as you can. Hold the position for about 10 seconds, feeling a stretch in your back, arms, and chest. Release your arms.

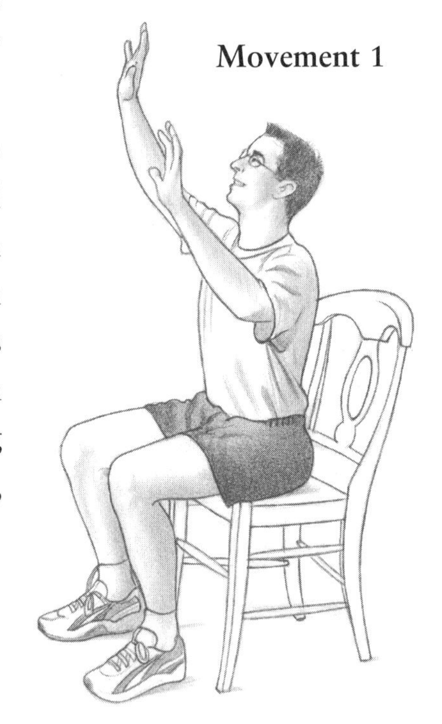

Movement 1

EXERCISE 4

Movement 3: Interlace your fingers in front of your body. Raise your arms so that they're parallel to the ground. Rotate your hands so your palms face an imaginary wall. Stand up straight, but curl your shoulders forward. You should feel the stretch in your wrists and upper back. Hold the position for about 10 seconds.

Repeat the exercise 3 times.

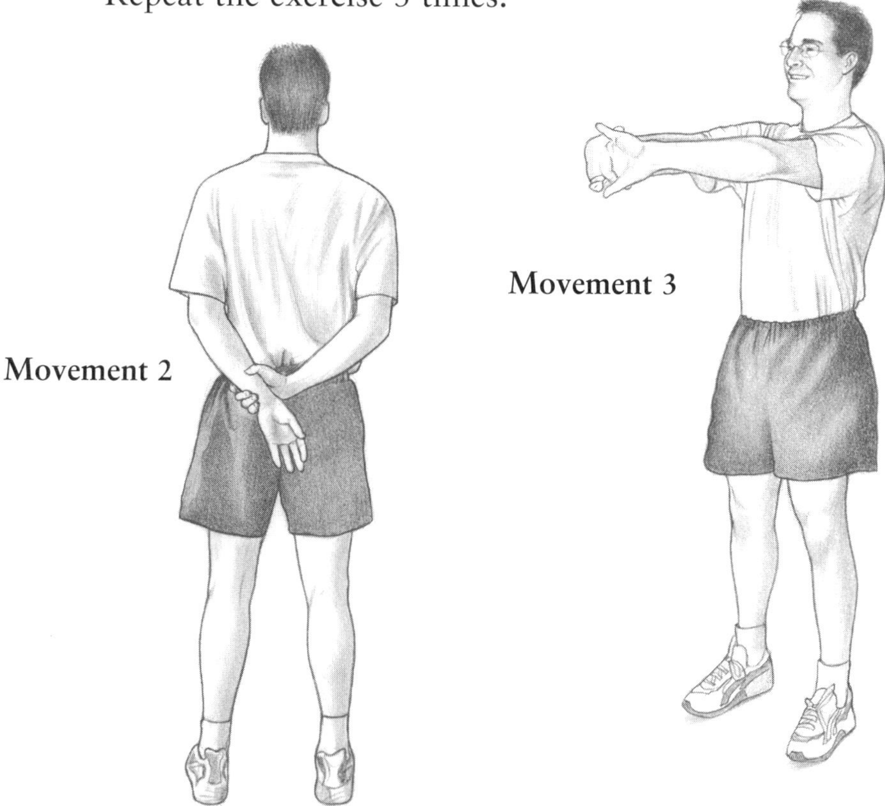

AFTER DOING PART I OF THE PROGRAM FOR 2 WEEKS, YOU'RE READY TO MOVE ON TO PART II.

GAINING GRIP STRENGTH

If you have arthritis, you may have trouble picking up things with your hands or keeping a grip on them. Some of the exercises in the next section of this book will help strengthen your hand muscles. If you're concerned about grip strength, you may also want to add a grip exercise to increase strength and decrease stiffness in your hands. The exercise is simple; it can be done easily while reading or watching TV, and most people already have the equipment at home.

Equipment: Racquetball, tennis ball, or "stress" ball.

Time: Less than 5 minutes.

Exercise: Grasp a ball in one hand while sitting or standing. Slowly squeeze it as hard as you can and hold the squeeze for 3 to 5 seconds. Slowly release the squeeze. Take a short rest, then repeat the exercise 10 times. Switch hands, and do 2 sets of 10 squeezes with the other hand.

Frequency: You may do this exercise every day or every other day, depending on how your hands feel. If they feel stiff or painful, you may want to skip a day.

PART II:

STEPPING UP YOUR STRENGTH

This part of the program is more challenging because it adds weights to the exercises. When you start this part, approach the exercises enthusiastically but with care. It's important to exercise at the proper intensity, with the correct amount of weight for your current level of strength. You are working at the right intensity (or difficulty) if you can complete 10 repetitions of a given exercise—and no more. Whatever your current level of strength, it is best to start this part using 2- to 3-pound weights for both dumbbells and ankle weights. This will reduce your risk of injury.

Exercise Tip

Don't perform the exercises quickly. They should be done in a slow, controlled motion.

EXERCISE 5

PART II:

STEPPING UP YOUR STRENGTH CONTINUED

Reassess the intensity of the exercises after completing one week (or 3 sessions) of each set of exercises. Start using heavier weights if any exercise seems easy with the weights you are using and you can complete more than 10 repetitions in proper form.

After a few weeks of these exercises, you'll find it easier to lift and carry heavy items, complete household chores, and walk distances without discomfort.

BICEPS CURL

Does a gallon of milk feel a lot heavier than it used to? After a few weeks of doing the biceps curl, lifting that eight-pound jug will be a cinch!

1. Stand or sit in a chair with a dumbbell in each hand. Your feet should be shoulder-width apart with your arms at your sides and your palms facing your thighs.
2. Rotate your forearms and slowly lift the weights as you count to 2. Your palms should be facing in towards your shoulders. Keep your upper arms and elbows close to your

EXERCISE 5

side—as if you had a newspaper tucked under your arm.

3. Pause. Then, slowly lower the dumbbells back towards your thighs as you count to four. Rotate your forearms so that your arms are again at your sides, palms facing your thighs.

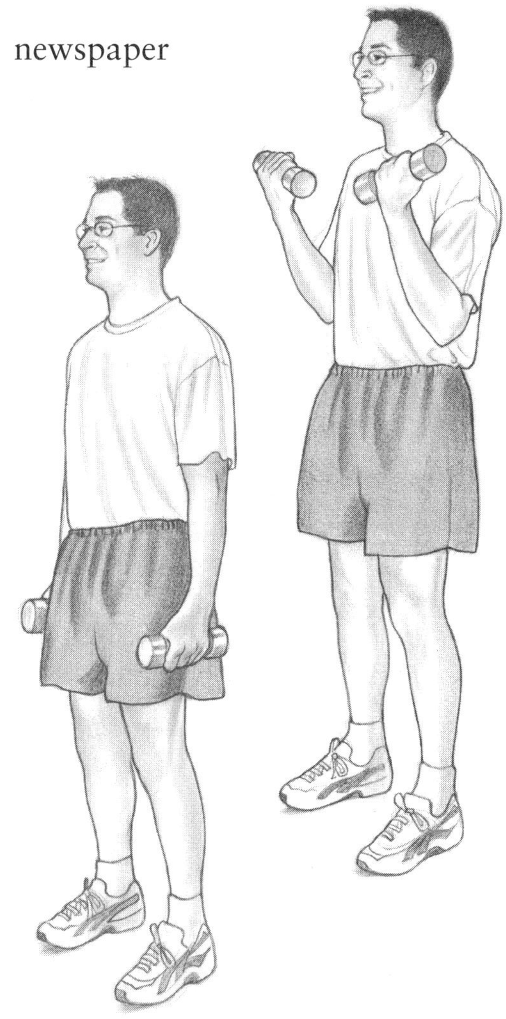

Repeat 10 times for 1 set. Rest for about 1 minute. Then complete a second set of 10 repetitions.

MAKE SURE YOU

Don't let your upper arms or elbows move away from the sides of your body.

Keep your wrists straight.

EXERCISE 6

STEP-UPS

This is a great strengthening exercise that requires only a set of stairs. But don't let its simplicity fool you. Step-ups will improve your balance and build strength in your legs, hips, and buttocks.

1. Stand next to a handrail at the bottom of a staircase. With your feet flat and toes facing forward, put your entire left foot on the first step.
2. Hold the handrail for balance. As you count to 2, place your weight on your left leg and straighten it as you slowly lift your right leg until it reaches the first step. Make sure that your left knee stays straight and does not move forward past your ankle as you're lifting yourself up. Let your right foot tap the first step near your left foot.
3. Pause. Then, use your left leg to support your weight and slowly lower your right foot back to the floor as you count to 4.

Repeat 10 times with the left leg and 10 times with the right leg for 1 set. Rest for about 1 minute. Then do a second set of 10 repetitions with each leg.

EXERCISE 6

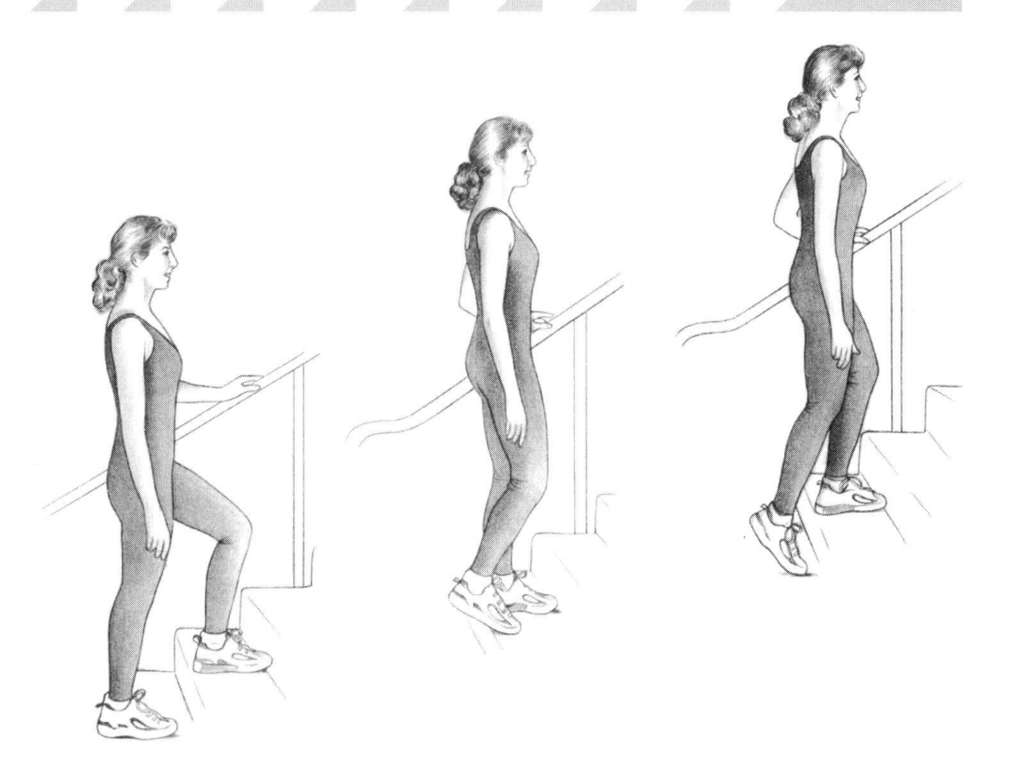

MAKE SURE YOU

Don't let your back leg do the work.

Don't let momentum do the work.

Press your weight on the heel rather than ball or toes of your front leg as you lift.

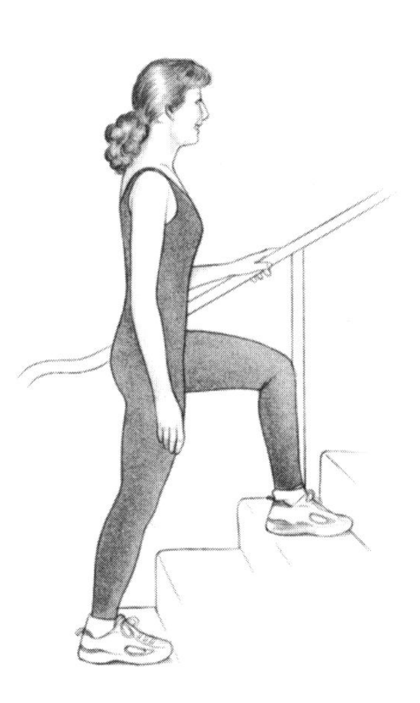

Advanced Move:

When you're ready, you can use 2 stairs rather than 1.

EXERCISE 7

OVERHEAD PRESS

This useful exercise targets several muscles in the arms, upper back, and shoulders. It can also help firm the back of your upper arms and make reaching for objects in high cupboards easier.

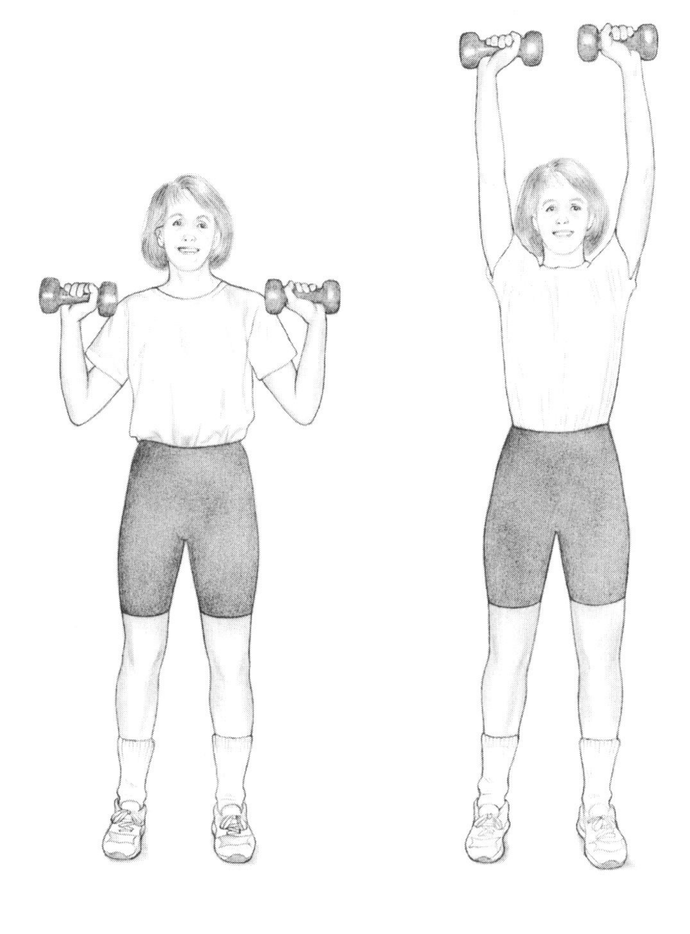

EXERCISE 7

1. Stand or sit in a chair with feet shoulder-width apart. Pick up a dumbbell in each hand. Raise your hands with your palms and forearms facing forward, until the dumbbells are level with your shoulders and parallel to the floor.
2. Slowly push the dumbbells up over your head until your arms are fully extended as you count to 2. Make sure you don't lock your elbows.
3. Pause. Then, slowly lower the dumbbells back to shoulder level as you count to 4, bringing your elbows down close to your sides.

Repeat 10 times for 1 set. Rest for about 1 minute. Then complete a second set of 10 repetitions.

MAKE SURE YOU

Keep your wrists straight.

Relax your neck and shoulders.

Don't lock your elbows; keep a slight bend in your arms.

Don't let the dumbbells move too far in front of your body or behind it.

Breathe regularly throughout the exercise.

EXERCISE 8

SIDE HIP RAISE

The side hip raise targets the muscles in your hips, thighs, and buttocks. This exercise firms and shapes your lower body, and strengthens your hipbones, which are more vulnerable to fracture as you age.

1. Stand behind a sturdy chair, with feet slightly apart and toes facing forward. Keep your legs straight, but do not lock your knees.
2. Slowly lift your left leg out to the side as you count to 2. Keep your leg straight—but again, do not lock your knee.
3. Pause. Then, slowly lower your left foot back to the ground as you count to 4.

Repeat 10 times with the left leg and 10 times with the right leg for 1 set. Rest for about 1 minute. Then do a second set of 10 repetitions with each leg.

Note

Only a small amount of movement out to the side is necessary. It is very important to do this exercise in a slow, controlled motion.

EXERCISE 8

MAKE SURE YOU:

Don't lock your knee on the supporting leg.

Keep your toes facing forward throughout the move.

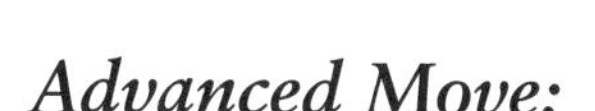

Advanced Move:

You may add ankle weights to make the exercise more difficult, as shown above. Start with 1 to 3 pounds.

AFTER YOU HAVE DONE THE EXERCISES IN PARTS I AND II OF THE PROGRAM 2 OR 3 TIMES A WEEK FOR AT LEAST 4 WEEKS, YOU ARE READY TO MOVE ON TO PART III.

EXERCISE 9

PART III:

COMPLEMENTING YOUR PROGRAM

The next exercises add variety to your routine and give you new ways to increase your strength. Exercises 9 and 10 target the muscles of the upper leg and require ankle weights. These exercises should be done together. Exercises 11 and 12 strengthen the abdomen and the back and should also be done together. As with all strength-training exercises, remember to breathe throughout each exercise. When you start to use ankle weights, use 1 to 3 pounds and increase the weight as you get stronger over time.

Exercise Tip

Never wear ankle weights or hold dumbbells while walking or doing other aerobic exercises such as biking or jogging.

EXERCISE 9

KNEE EXTENSION

This exercise strengthens weak knees and reduces the symptoms of arthritis of the knee by targeting the muscles of the front of the thigh.

1. Put your ankle weights on snugly. Sit all the way back in a sturdy chair so that your feet barely touch the ground. If your chair is too low, add a rolled-up towel under your knees.
2. Point your toes forward. Flex your left foot and slowly lift your left leg as you count to two. Extend your leg until your knee is straight.
3. Pause. Then, slowly lower your foot back to the ground as you count to 4.

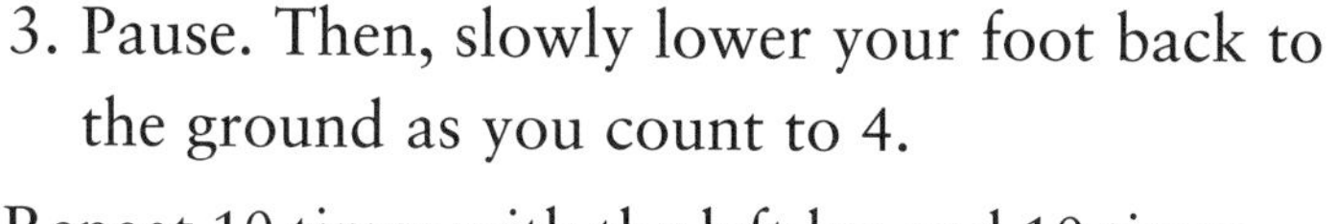

Repeat 10 times with the left leg and 10 times with the right leg for 1 set. Rest for 1 to 2 minutes. Then do a second set of 10 repetitions with each leg.

MAKE SURE YOU

Keep your ankle flexed throughout the move.

EXERCISE 10

KNEE CURL

This is an excellent exercise for strengthening the muscles of the back of the upper leg, known as the hamstrings. Walking and climbing are easier when you do both the knee extensions and knee curl.

1. Keep your ankle weights on and stand behind a sturdy chair. Your feet should be a little less than shoulder-width apart and face forward.
2. Keep your foot flexed and slowly bend your right leg and bring your heel up toward your buttocks as you count to 2.
3. Pause. Then, slowly lower your foot back to the ground as you count to 4.

Repeat 10 times with your right leg and 10 times with your left leg for one set. Rest for 1 to 2 minutes. Then do a second set of 10 repetitions with each leg.

EXERCISE 10

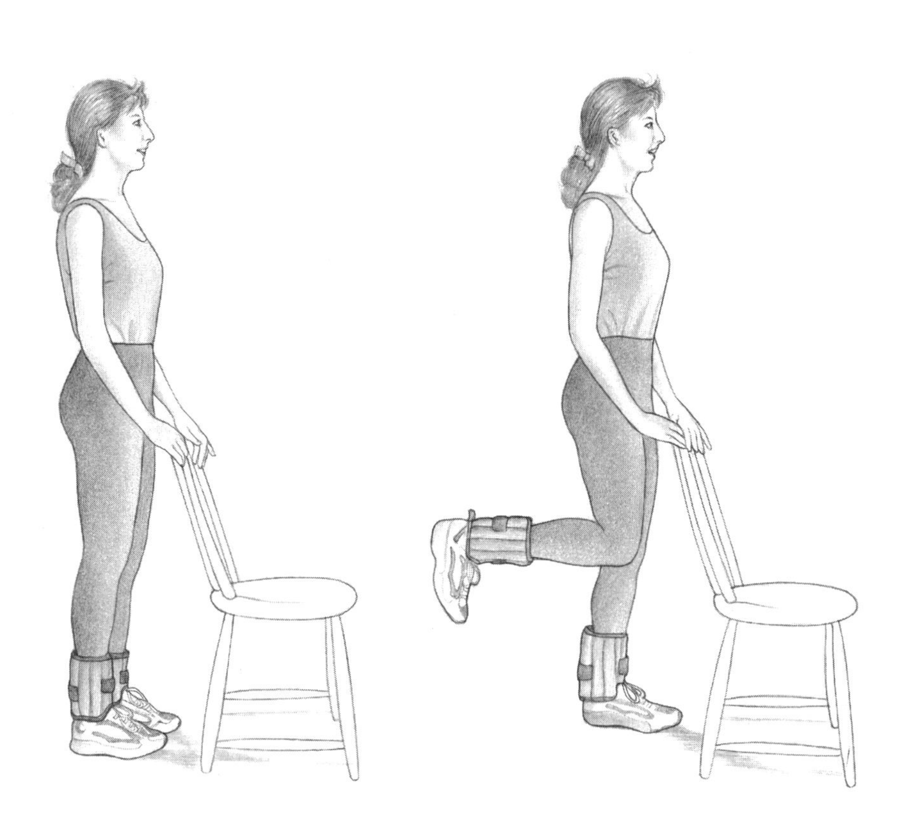

MAKE SURE YOU

Keep the thigh of the working leg in line with the supporting leg at all times.

Keep the foot of the working leg flexed throughout the move.

EXERCISE 11

PELVIC TILT

This exercise improves posture and tightens the muscles in your abdomen and buttocks. Do this exercise with the floor back extension—described next in Exercise 12—to strengthen your midsection. (You should not have the ankle weights on during this exercise.)

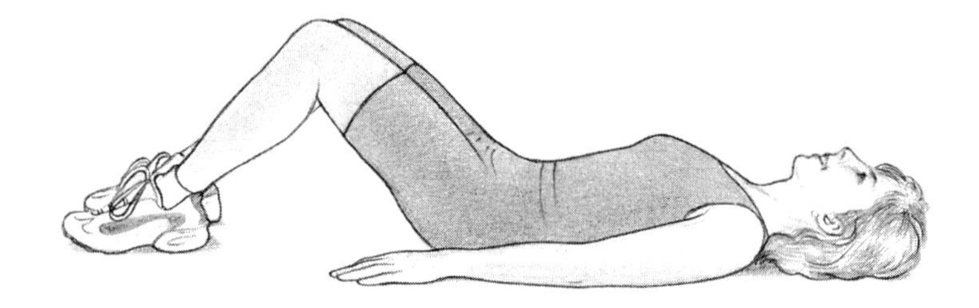

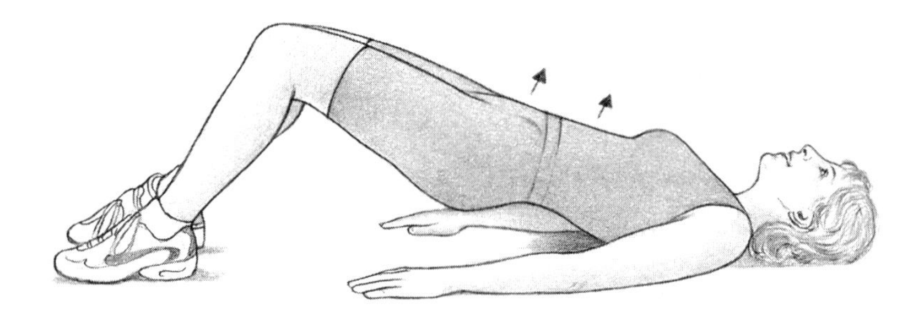

EXERCISE 11

1. Lie flat on your back on the floor or on a firm mattress. Keep your knees bent, feet flat, and arms at your sides. The palms of your hands should face the ground.
2. Slowly roll your pelvis toward your abdomen so that your hips and lower back are off the floor as you count to 2. Your upper back and shoulders should remain in place.
3. Pause. Then, slowly lower your pelvis all the way down as you count to 4.

Repeat 10 times for 1 set. Rest for 1 to 2 minutes. Then do a second set of 10 repetitions.

MAKE SURE YOU:

Breathe throughout the exercise.

Don't lift your upper back or shoulders off the ground.

EXERCISE 12

FLOOR BACK EXTENSION

You may suffer from lower back pain because your back muscles are weak. The floor back extension, done with the pelvic tilt, will strengthen these muscles and ease back pain.

1. Lie on the floor face-down. Extend your left arm straight overhead so that it aligns with your body. Keep the other arm at your side.
2. Slowly lift your left arm and right leg off the ground as you count to 2. Keep your arm and leg at the same level.
3. Pause. Then slowly lower your arm and leg back to the ground as you count to 4.

Repeat 10 times for 1 set, and then switch to the right arm and the left leg for another 10 repetitions. Rest for 1 to 2 minutes. Then, do a second set of 10 repetitions.

EXERCISE 12

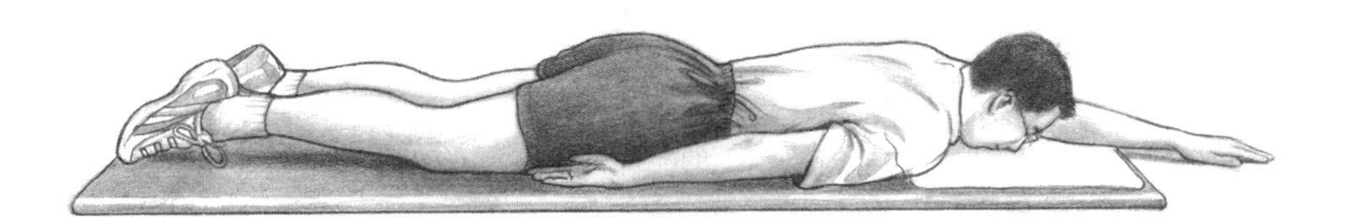

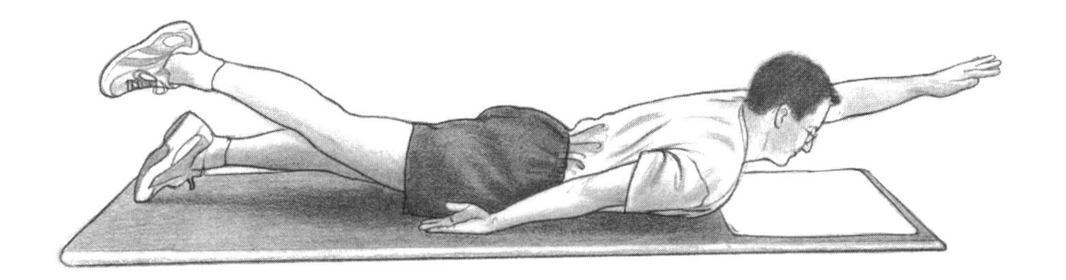

MAKE SURE YOU

Keep your head, neck, and back in a straight line.

COOL-DOWN

COOL-DOWN:

STRETCHING FOR FLEXIBILITY AND RELAXATION

Cooling down right after completing your workout is just as important as warming up before starting to exercise. Stretching is an excellent way to cool down, improve flexibility, and avoid injuries. It will also relieve tension and help you relax. In fact, it's a good idea to stretch and breathe deeply whenever you feel tense or need to relax—it will benefit your body and mind.

Do the following stretches after each strength-training workout, along with any others you already know.

Exercise Tip

Remember to hold the stretch for at least 20 to 30 seconds each time.

COOL-DOWN 1

CHEST AND ARM STRETCH

This simple reaching stretch will improve the flexibility in your arms and chest and in the front of your shoulders.

1. Stand with your arms at your sides and your feet about shoulder-width apart.
2. Extend both arms behind your back and clasp your hands together. Retract your shoulders if possible.
3. Hold the stretch for a slow count of 20 to 30 seconds, breathing throughout.

Release the stretch and repeat.

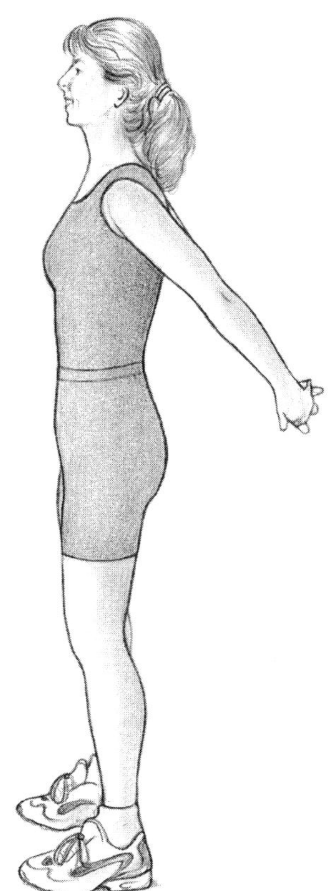

MAKE SURE YOU

Breathe throughout the stretch.

Keep your back straight, relax your shoulders, and look straight ahead.

COOL-DOWN 2

HAMSTRING/CALF STRETCH

If touching your toes with straight legs seems too difficult, you're not alone. Many people have tight muscles in the back of the leg. This stretch will give these muscles more flexibility and make it easier for you to bend and reach.

1. Stand facing a sturdy chair.
2. Slowly bend forward at the hip, keeping your legs straight without locking your knees. Rest your hands on the seat of the chair with your elbows slightly bent, feeling a stretch in the back of your upper and lower leg. Keep your back flat.
3. Hold the stretch for a slow count of 20 to 30 seconds, breathing throughout.

Release the stretch and repeat.

Note

If this stretch is too easy and you're not feeling a comfortable pull in the back of your legs, try bending your elbows more. Try going as far as to rest your forearms and elbows on the seat of the chair. Just make sure you are bending at the hips and keeping your back straight.

COOL-DOWN 2

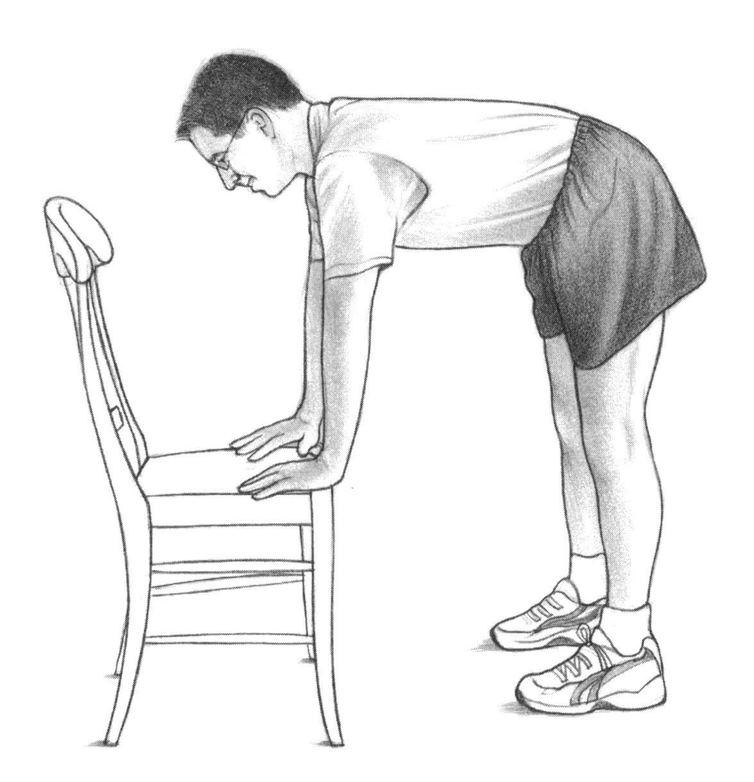

MAKE SURE YOU

Breathe throughout the stretch and concentrate on relaxing.

Keep your back straight as you bend towards the chair.

COOL-DOWN 3

QUADRICEPS STRETCH

This excellent stretch should be a regular part of your cool-down. Strength-training exercises such as squats, step-ups, and knee extensions focus on strengthening the quadriceps muscles. This stretch will help these muscles relax and make them more flexible.

1. Stand next to a counter or sturdy chair with your feet about shoulder-width apart and your knees straight—but not locked.
2. Hold a chair or counter for balance with your left hand. Bend your right leg back and grab your right foot or ankle in your right hand until your thigh is perpendicular to the ground. Make sure you stand up straight—don't lean forward. (If you can't grab your ankle in your hand, just keep your leg as close to perpendicular as possible and hold the bend.) You should feel a stretch in the front of your thigh.
3. Hold the stretch for a slow count of 20 to 30 seconds, breathing throughout.

Release your right ankle and repeat the stretch with the other leg.

COOL-DOWN 3

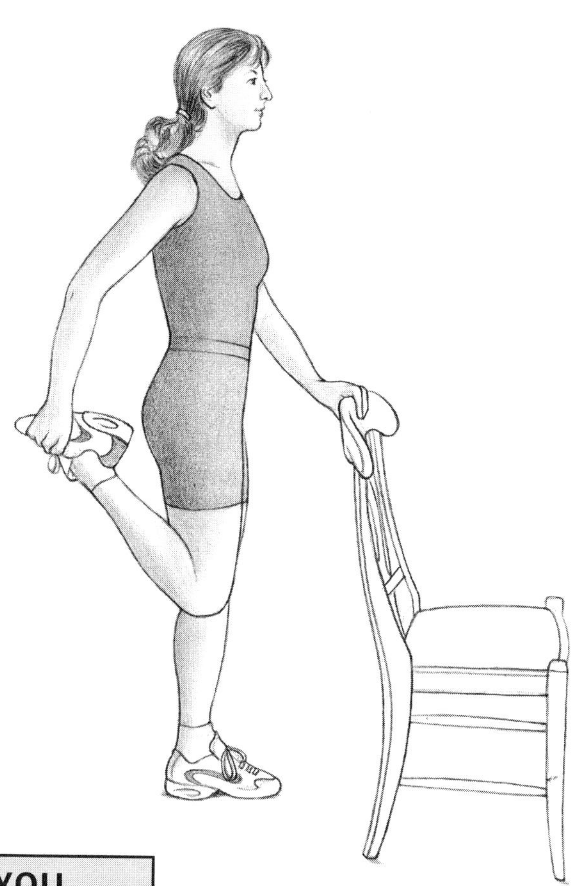

MAKE SURE YOU

Breathe throughout the stretch and concentrate on relaxing.

Stand up straight and look ahead.

Don't lock your supporting knee.

COOL-DOWN 4

NECK, UPPER BACK, AND SHOULDER STRETCH

This easy stretch targets another group of muscles that are easily tensed and stressed—the neck, back, and shoulders. Stretch after strength training and during any activity that makes you feel stiff, such as sitting at a desk. You'll find it will give you energy.

1. Stand (or sit) with your feet shoulder-width apart, your knees straight but not locked, and your hands clasped in front of you. Rotate your hands so that your palms face the ground. Then raise your arms to about chest height.
2. Press your palms away from your body and feel a stretch in your neck, upper back, and along your shoulders.
3. Hold the stretch for a slow count of 20 to 30 seconds, breathing throughout.

Release the stretch and repeat.

COOL-DOWN 4

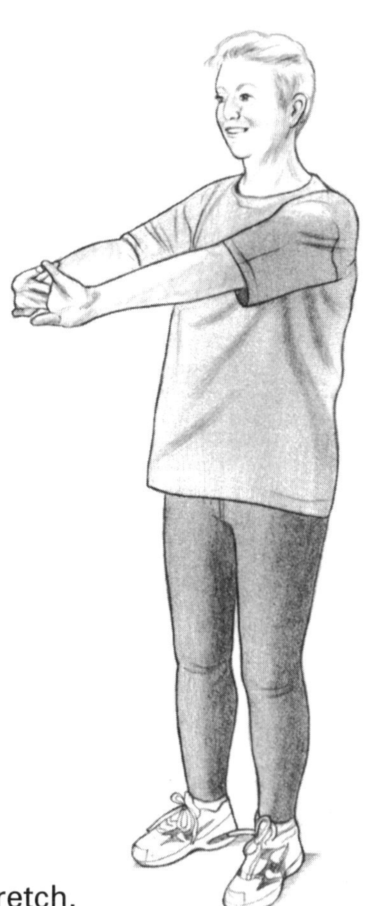

MAKE SURE YOU

Breathe throughout the stretch.

Don't curve or arch your back.

chapter 6

The Courage to Progress

Once you can do the exercises in Part III of the program, you will likely have gained a lot of muscle mass and strength and improved your balance, coordination, and flexibility. Congratulations. It's a great achievement to start and continue a strength-training program. It's important to progress if you want to experience the many benefits of strength training. This means always advancing the intensity of your workout by using heavier weights. As a result, your muscles will grow and stay strong. You will also feel more independent and will be more able to live well into old age without the fear of falling. It will also give you a great sense of pride and accomplishment.

HOW TO PROGRESS

After about the first week of strength training, you should start doing each exercise with weights that you can lift at least 10 times with only moderate difficulty. The weight you are using may be too heavy if you can't do a given exercise 8 times in a row. You may need to scale back.

You should rethink whether the weights you are using are heavy enough after 2 weeks of strength training. You may start doing the overhead press with 2-pound dumbbells, for example. By the end of the second week, you may be able to easily lift the 2-pound dumbbell more than 12 times. Make sure you are doing all the movements in the exercise and that your body is positioned properly (known as good form). You should now try to use 3-pound dumbbells and see how the exercise feels.

WHEN TO PROGRESS—AND WHEN NOT TO

It may be time to add heavier weights to your workout if you are in good health, are exercising regularly, and a given exercise feels too easy. An exercise should be considered too easy if you can do it more than 10 or 12 times with the weights you have currently been using. Do not progress if you have been sick, are injured, or your muscles feel very sore.

WORKING AT THE RIGHT INTENSITY—JUDGING YOUR EFFORT

It is important to find the right balance between being careful when exercising to prevent injury and always progressing to increase strength. This easy-to-use scale will help you find the right intensity for your workout.

EXERCISE INTENSITY INDICATOR

Ask Yourself These Questions After Each Exercise

1. Were you able to complete 2 sets of 10 repetitions in good form?

No — Reduce the weight so you can lift 10 times in good form; then repeat for a second set.

Yes — Please continue to question 2.

2. After completing 10 repetitions, do you need to rest because the weight is too heavy to complete more repetitions in good form?

Yes — You are working at the right intensity and should not increase the weight.

No — Please continue to questions three and four to determine how to safely increase the intensity of your workout.

EXERCISE INTENSITY INDICATOR
Continued

3. Could you have done a few more repetitions in good form without a break?

Yes — You may feel that you can do only a few more repetitions—not the entire next set of ten without a break. At your next workout, do the first set of repetitions with the current weight you have been using. Then do the second set with a slightly heavier weight. For example, if you're currently using 2-pound dumbbells, use 3-pound dumbbells for your second set.

4. Could you have done all twenty repetitions at one time, without a break?

Yes — Use heavier dumbbells for both sets of repetitions the next time you workout.

NOTE 1

Remember that you should complete each repetition in proper form, using the "2-up, pause, 4-down" count.

NOTE 2

When you start doing the exercises with the adjustable ankle weights, you will be able to increase intensity by adding half- or 1-pound weights to each leg.

chapter 7 Staying on Track: A 12-Week Workbook

It's important to stick to your strength-training program as much as you can. You may find that you make a few false starts before you succeed at making this program a regular part of your life. There may be times when interruptions such as vacation, illness, family, or work demands prevent you from doing your exercises for a week or 2—or even longer. Try not to feel guilty or disappointed in yourself. Just restart your routine as quickly as you can. You may not be able to pick up exactly where you left off—you may need to decrease your weights a bit. But stay with it, and you will regain lost ground.

If you have trouble getting back into the swing of things, start back into the program slowly. Remember why you picked up this book in the first place and why you chose your goals. It may help to reassess your goals and make new ones because your motivations may change as time passes. Most important, remember how your past successes made you feel: healthy, strong, independent, and empowered!

You'll find a workbook on the following pages with a 12-week supply of easy-to-use exercise log sheets. Each log sheet has a motivational or instructional tip. At the end of the 12-week supply, you will find a blank log sheet for photocopying so you can keep track of your progress. These log sheets will help you accurately monitor your progress in strength training. Keeping a record in this workbook is an important part of the program and will help you succeed.

WEEK 1 Date:

LOG SHEET

EXERCISES	DAY 1	DAY 2	DAY 3
2 Sets of 10 Repetitions	**WEIGHT LIFTED OR CHECK (√) WHEN EXERCISE IS COMPLETED.**		
SQUATS			
WALL PUSH-UPS			
TOE STANDS			
FINGER MARCHING			
STRETCHES	**CHECK WHEN COMPLETED**		
Hold for 20–30 Seconds			
CHEST & ARMS			
HAMSTRINGS			
QUADRICEPS			
NECK AND BACK			

WEEK 1

Count out loud during the exercises to make sure you keep the proper pace.

Personal Notes

RECORD ANY ADDITIONAL ACTIVITIES/EXERCISES HERE

ACTIVITY	DESCRIPTION
Hiking	*1 hour, felt energized*

WEEK 2 Date:

LOG SHEET

EXERCISES	DAY 1	DAY 2	DAY 3
2 Sets of 10 Repetitions	**WEIGHT LIFTED OR CHECK (√) WHEN EXERCISE IS COMPLETED.**		
SQUATS			
WALL PUSH-UPS			
TOE STANDS			
FINGER MARCHING			

STRETCHES	CHECK WHEN COMPLETED		
Hold for 20–30 Seconds			
CHEST & ARMS			
HAMSTRINGS			
QUADRICEPS			
NECK AND BACK			

WEEK 2

Strength training 2 or 3 times a week will help prevent arthritis and/or ease its symptoms.

Personal Notes

RECORD ANY ADDITIONAL ACTIVITIES/EXERCISES HERE

ACTIVITY	DESCRIPTION

WEEK 3 Date:

LOG SHEET

EXERCISES	DAY 1	DAY 2	DAY 3
2 Sets of 10 Repetitions	**WEIGHT LIFTED OR CHECK (√) WHEN EXERCISE IS COMPLETED.**		
SQUATS			
WALL PUSH-UPS			
TOE STANDS			
FINGER MARCHING			
BICEPS CURL			
STEP-UPS			
OVERHEAD PRESS			
SIDE HIP RAISE			
STRETCHES	**CHECK WHEN COMPLETED**		
Hold for 20–30 Seconds			
CHEST & ARMS			
HAMSTRINGS			
QUADRICEPS			
NECK AND BACK			

WEEK 3

Breathe throughout each exercise.

Personal Notes

RECORD ANY ADDITIONAL ACTIVITIES/EXERCISES HERE

ACTIVITY	DESCRIPTION

WEEK 4 Date:

LOG SHEET

EXERCISES	DAY 1	DAY 2	DAY 3
2 Sets of 10 Repetitions	**WEIGHT LIFTED OR CHECK (√) WHEN EXERCISE IS COMPLETED.**		
SQUATS			
WALL PUSH-UPS			
TOE STANDS			
FINGER MARCHING			
BICEPS CURL			
STEP-UPS			
OVERHEAD PRESS			
SIDE HIP RAISE			
STRETCHES	**CHECK WHEN COMPLETED**		
Hold for 20–30 Seconds			
CHEST & ARMS			
HAMSTRINGS			
QUADRICEPS			
NECK AND BACK			

WEEK 4

Strength training will make you feel energized!

Personal Notes

RECORD ANY ADDITIONAL ACTIVITIES/EXERCISES HERE

ACTIVITY	DESCRIPTION

WEEK 5 Date:

LOG SHEET

EXERCISES	DAY 1	DAY 2	DAY 3
2 Sets of 10 Repetitions	**WEIGHT LIFTED OR CHECK (√) WHEN EXERCISE IS COMPLETED.**		
SQUATS			
WALL PUSH-UPS			
TOE STANDS			
FINGER MARCHING			
BICEPS CURL			
STEP-UPS			
OVERHEAD PRESS			
HIP ABDUCTION			
STRETCHES	**CHECK WHEN COMPLETED**		
Hold for 20–30 Seconds			
CHEST & ARMS			
HAMSTRINGS			
QUADRICEPS			
NECK AND BACK			

WEEK 5

Look in a mirror to make sure that your form matches what is shown in the picture.

Personal Notes

RECORD ANY ADDITIONAL ACTIVITIES/EXERCISES HERE

ACTIVITY	DESCRIPTION

WEEK 6 Date:

LOG SHEET

EXERCISES	DAY 1	DAY 2	DAY 3
2 Sets of 10 Repetitions	**WEIGHT LIFTED OR CHECK (√) WHEN EXERCISE IS COMPLETED.**		
SQUATS			
WALL PUSH-UPS			
TOE STANDS			
FINGER MARCHING			
BICEPS CURL			
STEP-UPS			
OVERHEAD PRESS			
SIDE HIP RAISE			

STRETCHES	CHECK WHEN COMPLETED		
Hold for 20–30 Seconds			
CHEST & ARMS			
HAMSTRINGS			
QUADRICEPS			
NECK AND BACK			

WEEK 6

When you can do more than 10 repetitions in good form, increase the weight you are lifting.

Personal Notes

RECORD ANY ADDITIONAL ACTIVITIES/EXERCISES HERE

ACTIVITY	DESCRIPTION

WEEK 7 Date:

LOG SHEET

EXERCISES	DAY 1	DAY 2	DAY 3
2 Sets of 10 Repetitions	**WEIGHT LIFTED OR CHECK (√) WHEN EXERCISE IS COMPLETED.**		
SQUATS			
WALL PUSH-UPS			
TOE STANDS			
FINGER MARCHING			
BICEPS CURL			
STEP-UPS			
OVERHEAD PRESS			
SIDE HIP RAISE			
KNEE EXTENSION			
KNEE CURL			
PELVIC TILT			
BACK EXTENSION			
STRETCHES	**CHECK WHEN COMPLETED**		
Hold for 20–30 Seconds			
CHEST & ARMS			
HAMSTRINGS			
QUADRICEPS			
NECK AND BACK			

WEEK 7

Strength training will help you build and maintain strong bones.

Personal Notes

RECORD ANY ADDITIONAL ACTIVITIES/EXERCISES HERE

ACTIVITY	DESCRIPTION

WEEK 8 Date:

LOG SHEET

EXERCISES	DAY 1	DAY 2	DAY 3
2 Sets of 10 Repetitions	**WEIGHT LIFTED OR CHECK (√) WHEN EXERCISE IS COMPLETED.**		
SQUATS			
WALL PUSH-UPS			
TOE STANDS			
FINGER MARCHING			
BICEPS CURL			
STEP-UPS			
OVERHEAD PRESS			
SIDE HIP RAISE			
KNEE EXTENSION			
KNEE CURL			
PELVIC TILT			
BACK EXTENSION			
STRETCHES	**CHECK WHEN COMPLETED**		
Hold for 20–30 Seconds			
CHEST & ARMS			
HAMSTRINGS			
QUADRICEPS			
NECK AND BACK			

WEEK 8

Strength training will help you sleep better.

Personal Notes

RECORD ANY ADDITIONAL ACTIVITIES/EXERCISES HERE

ACTIVITY	DESCRIPTION

WEEK 9 Date:

LOG SHEET

EXERCISES	DAY 1	DAY 2	DAY 3
2 Sets of 10 Repetitions	**WEIGHT LIFTED OR CHECK (√) WHEN EXERCISE IS COMPLETED.**		
SQUATS			
WALL PUSH-UPS			
TOE STANDS			
FINGER MARCHING			
BICEPS CURL			
STEP-UPS			
OVERHEAD PRESS			
SIDE HIP RAISE			
KNEE EXTENSION			
KNEE CURL			
PELVIC TILT			
BACK EXTENSION			
STRETCHES	**CHECK WHEN COMPLETED**		
Hold for 20–30 Seconds			
CHEST & ARMS			
HAMSTRINGS			
QUADRICEPS			
NECK AND BACK			

WEEK 9

During squats and step-ups, make sure that your knees don't move forward past your toes.

Personal Notes

RECORD ANY ADDITIONAL ACTIVITIES/EXERCISES HERE

ACTIVITY	DESCRIPTION

WEEK 10 Date:

LOG SHEET

EXERCISES	DAY 1	DAY 2	DAY 3
2 Sets of 10 Repetitions	**WEIGHT LIFTED OR CHECK (√) WHEN EXERCISE IS COMPLETED.**		
SQUATS			
WALL PUSH-UPS			
TOE STANDS			
FINGER MARCHING			
BICEPS CURL			
STEP-UPS			
OVERHEAD PRESS			
SIDE HIP RAISE			
KNEE EXTENSION			
KNEE CURL			
PELVIC TILT			
BACK EXTENSION			
STRETCHES	**CHECK WHEN COMPLETED**		
Hold for 20–30 Seconds			
CHEST & ARMS			
HAMSTRINGS			
QUADRICEPS			
NECK AND BACK			

WEEK 10

Strength training will make aerobic exercise such as swimming, biking, and walking easier.

Personal Notes

RECORD ANY ADDITIONAL ACTIVITIES/EXERCISES HERE

ACTIVITY	DESCRIPTION

WEEK 11 Date:

LOG SHEET

EXERCISES	DAY 1	DAY 2	DAY 3
2 Sets of 10 Repetitions	**WEIGHT LIFTED OR CHECK (√) WHEN EXERCISE IS COMPLETED.**		
SQUATS			
WALL PUSH-UPS			
TOE STANDS			
FINGER MARCHING			
BICEPS CURL			
STEP-UPS			
OVERHEAD PRESS			
SIDE HIP RAISE			
KNEE EXTENSION			
KNEE CURL			
PELVIC TILT			
BACK EXTENSION			
STRETCHES	**CHECK WHEN COMPLETED**		
Hold for 20–30 Seconds			
CHEST & ARMS			
HAMSTRINGS			
QUADRICEPS			
NECK AND BACK			

WEEK 11

During the biceps curl and overhead press, be sure to keep your wrists straight.

Personal Notes

RECORD ANY ADDITIONAL ACTIVITIES/EXERCISES HERE

ACTIVITY	DESCRIPTION

WEEK 12 Date:

LOG SHEET

EXERCISES	DAY 1	DAY 2	DAY 3
2 Sets of 10 Repetitions	**WEIGHT LIFTED OR CHECK (√) WHEN EXERCISE IS COMPLETED.**		
SQUATS			
WALL PUSH-UPS			
TOE STANDS			
FINGER MARCHING			
BICEPS CURL			
STEP-UPS			
OVERHEAD PRESS			
SIDE HIP RAISE			
KNEE EXTENSION			
KNEE CURL			
PELVIC TILT			
BACK EXTENSION			
STRETCHES	**CHECK WHEN COMPLETED**		
Hold for 20–30 Seconds			
CHEST & ARMS			
HAMSTRINGS			
QUADRICEPS			
NECK AND BACK			

WEEK 12

Strength training will help you maintain your independence.

Personal Notes

RECORD ANY ADDITIONAL ACTIVITIES/EXERCISES HERE

ACTIVITY	DESCRIPTION

FOR COPYING

WEEK Date:

LOG SHEET

EXERCISES	DAY 1	DAY 2	DAY 3
2 Sets of 10 Repetitions	**WEIGHT LIFTED OR CHECK (√) WHEN EXERCISE IS COMPLETED.**		
SQUATS			
WALL PUSH-UPS			
TOE STANDS			
FINGER MARCHING			
BICEPS CURL			
STEP-UPS			
OVERHEAD PRESS			
SIDE HIP RAISE			
KNEE EXTENSION			
KNEE CURL			
PELVIC TILT			
BACK EXTENSION			
STRETCHES	**CHECK WHEN COMPLETED**		
Hold for 20–30 Seconds			
CHEST & ARMS			
HAMSTRINGS			
QUADRICEPS			
NECK AND BACK			

WEEK

You can do it!

Personal Notes

RECORD ANY ADDITIONAL ACTIVITIES/EXERCISES HERE

ACTIVITY	DESCRIPTION

Resources for Staying Strong

ORGANIZATIONS

American Council on Exercise
4851 Paramount Drive, San Diego, CA 92123
(800) 825-3636 *www.acefitness.org*
A fitness organization that helps you locate certified exercise professionals in your area.

American College of Sports Medicine
P.O. Box 1440, Indianapolis, IN 46206
www.acsm.org
An organization that conducts research in the field of exercise science and certifies fitness professionals.

American Dietetics Association (ADA)
216 West Jackson Boulevard, Chicago, IL 60606-6995
(800) 366-1655 *www.eatright.org*
Features comprehensive nutrition information for the public, including a database of dieticians in your area.

Arthritis Foundation
P.O. Box 7669, Atlanta, GA 30357-0669
(800) 283-7800 *www.arthritis.org*
Comprehensive information for preventing and treating arthritis.

Centers for Disease Control and Prevention
National Center for Chronic Disease Prevention and Health Promotion (NCCDPHP); Division of Nutrition and Physical Activity (DNPA) *www.cdc.gov/nccdphp/dnpa*
4770 Buford Highway, NE, Atlanta, GA 30341-3717
Comprehensive information about nutrition, physical activity, and numerous other health-related topics.

John Hancock Center for Physical Activity and Nutrition
Friedman School of Nutrition Science and Policy at Tufts University
150 Harrison Avenue, Boston, MA 02111
www.nutrition.tufts.edu
Comprehensive information about nutrition, physical activity, and numerous other health-related topics.

Fifty-Plus Fitness Association
P.O. Box 20230, Stanford, CA 94309
(650) 323-6160 *www.50plus.org*
A national organization whose sole mission is the promotion of physical activity for older adults.

National Strength and Conditioning Association
1640 L Street, Suite G, Lincoln, NE 68508
(888) 746-2378 *www.nsca-lift.org*
An organization where you can locate certified fitness professionals in your geographical area.

National Osteoporosis Foundation
1150 17th Street N.W., Suite 500. Washington, DC 20036
(202) 223-2226 *www.nof.org*
Comprehensive information for preventing and treating osteoporosis.

Shape-Up America!
6707 Democracy Boulevard, Suite 306, Bethesda, MD 20817
(301) 493-5368 *www.shapeup.org*
Comprehensive information about nutrition, physical activity, and numerous other health-related topics.

BOOKS

Strong Women and Men Beat Arthritis, Miriam Nelson, Kristin Baker, Ronenn Roubenoff, and Lawrence Lindner (Putnam, 2002).

Exercise: A Guide from the National Institute on Aging, Public Information Office. National Institutes of Health. Publication No. NIH 99-4258, June 2001.

Strong Women, Strong Bones, Miriam Nelson and Sarah Wernick (Putnam, 2000).

Strength Training Past 50, by Wayne Wescott, Thomas Baechler, and Mark Williams (Human Kinetics, 1997).

The Wellness Guide to Lifelong Fitness, by Timothy P. White, and the editors of the University of California at Berkeley Wellness Letter (Rebus, 1993).

Biomarkers: The 10 Determinants of Aging You Can Control, by William Evans, Irwin Rosenberg, and Jaqueline Thompson (Simon & Schuster, 1991).

EQUIPMENT CHECKLIST

BASIC:

- Sturdy chair
- Exercise space
- Rubber sole shoes
- Loose, comfortable clothing
- Dumbbells (hand-held weights)
- Adjustable ankle weights
- Stairs or raised platform
- Storage container

OPTIONAL:

- Rolling storage cart
- Mirror
- Heavier sets of dumbbells

Glossary

AEROBIC EXERCISE is physical activity that elevates the heart rate and breathing rate, thereby stimulating the cardiovascular system.

ARTHRITIS is the inflammation of a joint.

OSTEOARTHRITIS is the most common type of arthritis and is characterized by a degenerative process with inflammation around the joint.

RHEUMATOID ARTHRITIS is the most common type of inflammatory arthritis and usually affects many joints, including the hands and feet.

COOL-DOWN is the process of reducing the intensity of exercise at the end of a workout to help the body return to resting levels.

DURATION is the amount of time you spend doing a given exercise, whether it is aerobic exercise or strength training.

FREQUENCY defines how often you do the exercise; for example: three times each week.

INFLAMMATION is defined as pain, swelling, and redness caused by immune cells in response to injury or autoimmune disease.

INTENSITY (in the case of strength training) refers to the amount of weight you are lifting and indicates how difficult the exercise is for you to complete. Increasing your intensity (the weight you are lifting) is the key to progression and your success with a strength-training program.

OSTEOPOROSIS is a dangerous thinning of the bones that can increase a person's risk of fracture with minimal or little trauma.

REPETITION or "rep" refers to doing an exercise once through the complete range of motion. For instance, 1 push-up or 1 sit-up is a repetition.

SET is a group of repetitions completed consecutively. Typically, there are 8 to 12 repetitions in a set. There should always be a 1- to 2-minute rest between sets. Usually 1 to 3 sets are performed for a particular exercise.

STRENGTH TRAINING is an activity in which the muscle is working against a force such as a dumbbell, an ankle weight, or gravity. The intensity should be enough to increase muscular strength over time.

WARM-UP is the process of slowly increasing activity level and intensity prior to a workout to prepare the body for exercise.

Index

About the Authors

REBECCA A. SEGUIN, M.S., CSCS

Rebecca Seguin is Project Manager for the John Hancock Center for Physical Activity and Nutrition (JHCPAN) at the Gerald J. and Dorothy R. Friedman School of Nutrition Science and Policy at Tufts University in Boston. She received her bachelor's degree in Clinical Exercise Physiology from Boston University and her master's degree in Nutrition Communication from Tufts University. She has experience developing exercise programs for older adults and regularly writes exercise and nutrition articles for professional and lay press publications. She is certified by the National Strength and Conditioning Association (NSCA) as a Strength and Conditioning Specialist (CSCS) and is currently pursuing her doctoral degree at Tufts University.

JACQUELINE N. EPPING, M.ED.

Jacqueline Epping is a Public Health Educator in the Physical Activity and Health Branch, Division of Nutrition and Physical Activity, National Center for Chronic Disease Prevention and Health Promotion, U. S. Centers for Disease Control and Prevention. Ms. Epping has developed, implemented, and evaluated curricula and instructional materials for a number of studies to promote physical activity. She currently provides technical assistance to several national projects promoting physical activity in older adults.

DAVID M. BUCHNER, M.D., M.P.H.

David Buchner is Chief of the Physical Activity and Health Branch, Division of Nutrition and Physical Activity, National Center for Chronic Disease Prevention and Health Promotion, U. S. Centers for Disease Control and Prevention. With a specialty in geriatric medicine, Dr. Buchner has published extensively in the areas of physical activity in older adults and the role of physical activity in preventing fall injuries. He is the designer of the national award winning "Lifetime Fitness" exercise program, which has been disseminated in multiple centers throughout the state of Washington.

RINA BLOCH, M.D.

Rina Bloch is an Assistant Professor in the Department of Physical Medicine and Rehabilitation at Tufts University School of Medicine in Boston. She is an attending physician at Tufts-New England Medical Center.

MIRIAM E. NELSON, PH.D.

Miriam Nelson is Director of the John Hancock Center for Physical Activity and Nutrition (JHCPAN) at the Gerald J. and Dorothy R. Friedman School of Nutrition Science and Policy at Tufts University in Boston. She has been principal investigator on numerous studies of exercise and nutrition for older adults. Dr. Nelson is author of the internationally best selling *Strong Women* book series.